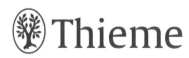

Radiology Structured Reporting Handbook

Disease-Specific Templates and Interpretation Pearls

Olga R. Brook, MD
Associate Professor
Harvard Medical School
Section Chief of Abdominal Radiology
Department of Radiology
Beth Israel Deaconess Medical Center
Boston, Massachusetts, USA

Wieland H. Sommer, MD, MPH
Professor of Radiology
Ludwig Maximilians University
Munich, Germany

266 illustrations

Thieme
New York • Stuttgart • Delhi • Rio de Janeiro

Library of Congress Cataloging-in-Publication Data
is available with the publisher.

© 2021 Thieme. All rights reserved.

Thieme Medical Publishers, Inc.
333 Seventh Avenue, 18th Floor
New York, NY 10001, USA
www.thieme.com
+1 800 782 3488, customerservice@thieme.com

Cover design: Thieme Publishing Group
Typesetting by DiTech Process Solutions, India

Printed in USA by King Printing Company, Inc.   5 4 3 2 1

ISBN 978-1-68420-151-8

Also available as an e-book:
eISBN 978-1-68420-152-5

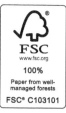

FSC
www.fsc.org
100%
Paper from well-managed forests
FSC® C103101

Contents

Contents

Section III Structured Reports in Abdominal Imaging

Editor: Olga R. Brook

Contents

Preface

"Analysis of a serum sample, and whole blood on citrate and EDTA. We compare the results to those of December 20th. We observe a slight rise in blood glucose level, but the value is still within normal limits. Erythrocytes sedimentate at a rather fair rate of 25 millimeters per hour, which can be considered just mildly abnormal, taking into account the patient's gender and age…"

This is the beginning of an article by Jan Bosmans et al entitled *Structured reporting: a fusion reactor hungry for fuel.*[1] The authors start with the prose transcription of the results of biochemical and hematological tests. Everyone expects these results in a neat and tabular manner. It appears unreasonable to describe these tests in a free-text form. However, in radiology, over the last 20 years, we have seen there is a long and heated debate, whether structured reporting is necessary, what are its advantages and disadvantages, and how it can be implemented.

This debate is supported by an exponential number of publications and conference presentations on the value and implementation of structured reporting in recent years (► Fig. 1).

Multiple studies show that referring physicians have a clear preference for structured reports due to their clarity and ease of interpretation, similar to the lab reports. However, there remains some resistance among radiologists to the structured reporting concept. The main concerns are usually due to the distraction from images by complex templates and splitting of complex pathologies into pre-defined simplistic subsections. We agree that simple structured reporting that contains subsections for visceral organs and vessels is not appropriate for complex studies. In complex cases, disease-specific structured reports would provide a better solution. Disease-specific structured reports are specifically tailored to the problem and also provide a checklist for radiologists of terms needed for clinical and surgical management of the specific problem.

This book contains disease-specific templates on the variety of conditions of neurological, cardiovascular, thoracic and abdominal diseases, and cancers. We have provided downloadable templates that can be directly implemented into the dictation program. Furthermore, specialists in corresponding fields have

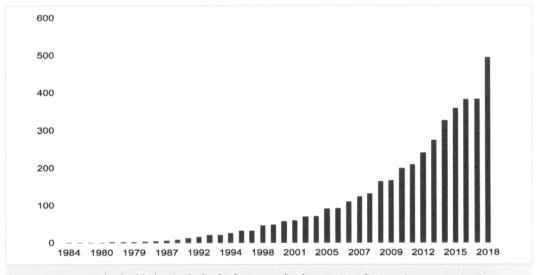

Fig. 1 Recent articles highlight the lack of information leading to a quality gap in communication.

provided list of pearls essential for interpretation of the specific study. Templates and pearls provide brief but to-the-point educational tool for trainees and senior people who do not interpret that specific type of study on a day-to-day basis.

Whereas the standardized display of biochemical and hematological tests is common sense for many decades, the field of radiology is currently undergoing a big change from "the art of imaging" to real data science. The standardization of the reporting is one of the first but essential steps in this transformation.

Olga R. Brook, MD
Wieland H. Sommer, MD, MPH

Reference

[1] Jan Bosmans et al. Structured reporting: a fusion reactor hungry for fuel. Insights imaging. 2015 Feb; 6(1): 129–32

Contributors

Lukas Abraszek, MD
Assistant
Department of Endocrine Oncology and Nuclear
    Medicine
Maria Sklodowska-Curie National Research Institute
    of Oncology
Warsaw, Poland

Muneeb Ahmed, MD, FSIR
Section Chief
Vascular and Interventional Radiology
Department of Radiology
Beth Israel Deaconess Medical Center
Boston, Massachusetts, USA

Ashley Hawk Aiken, MD
Director of Head and Neck Imaging
Program Director
Neuroradiology Fellowship
Professor
Department of Radiology and Imaging Sciences and
    Department of Otolaryngology–Head and Neck
    Surgery
Emory University School of Medicine
Atlanta, Georgia, USA

Tarik K. Alkasab, MD, PhD
Associate Chair
Enterprise Informatics/IT
Department of Radiology
Massachusetts General Hospital and Harvard Medical
    School
Boston, Massachusetts, USA

Jeff Ames, MD
Diagnostic Radiology Fellow
Department of Radiology
University of Minnesota
Minneapolis, Minnesota, USA

Thomas J.T. Anderson, MD
Assistant Professor
Department of Radiology
University of Massachusetts Medical School Baystate
Springfield, Massachusetts, USA

Regina G.H. Beets-Tan, MD, PhD
Radiologist and Head of Department
Department of Radiology
The Netherlands Cancer Institute
Amsterdam, the Netherlands

Hernan R. Bello, MD
Abdominal Radiology Fellow
Department of Radiology and Imaging Sciences
Emory University School of Medicine
Atlanta, Georgia, USA

Bernardo C. Bizzo, MD, MSc
Director, AI CRO
Department of Radiology
Massachusetts General Hospital, Harvard Medical
    School
Boston, Massachusetts, USA

Renata Rocha de Almeida Bizzo, MD, PhD
Clinical Fellow
Abdominal Imaging and Intervention
Brigham and Women's Hospital
Harvard Medical School
Boston, Massachusetts, USA

Olga R. Brook, MD
Associate Professor
Harvard Medical School
Section Chief of Abdominal Radiology
Department of Radiology
Beth Israel Deaconess Medical Center
Boston, Massachusetts, USA

Ricardo P. J. Budde, MD, PhD
Department of Radiology and Nuclear Medicine
Erasmus MC
Rotterdam, the Netherlands

Brett W. Carter, MD
Director of Clinical Operations
Chief Patient Safety and Quality Officer
Diagnostic Imaging
Associate Professor
Thoracic Imaging
MD Anderson Cancer Center
Houston, Texas, USA

Anne Catherine Kim, MD
Regional Lead
Stroke Imaging
Radiology
Kaiser Permanente Northern California
Walnut Creek, California, USA

Victoria Chernyak, MD, MS, FSAR
Professor of Radiology and Urology
Interim Section Chief
Division of Abdominal Imaging
Director of Body MR Imaging
Department of Radiology
Montefiore Medical Center
Bronx, New York, USA

Charlotte Y. Chung, MD, PhD
Diagnostic Radiology Resident
Department of Radiology and Imaging Sciences
Emory University School of Medicine
Atlanta, Georgia, USA

Jonathan H. Chung, MD
Associate Professor
Chief Quality Officer
Department of Radiology
Section Chief
Thoracic Radiology
The University of Chicago Medicine
Chicago, Illinois, USA

Francesca Coppola, MD
Consultant Radiologist
Malpighi Radiology Unit
S. Orsola-Malpighi University Hospital
Bologna, Italy

Elizabeth V. Craig, MD
Radiologist
Department of Radiology
Aurora St. Luke's Medical Center
Milwaukee, Wisconsin, USA

Mary Frances Croake, DO
Fellow
Department of Imaging Sciences
University of Rochester
Rochester, New York, USA

Nicole E. Curci, MD
Assistant Professor
Radiology
Michigan Medicine/University of Michigan
Ann Arbor, Michigan, USA

Jean-Nicolas Dacher, MD, PhD
Department of Radiology
Normandie University
UNIROUEN, INSERM U1096–Rouen University
   Hospital
Rouen, France

Matthew S. Davenport, MD, FSAR, FSABI
Associate Professor of Radiology and Urology
Department of Radiology
Michigan Medicine
Ann Arbor, Michigan, USA

Julien Dinkel, MD
Department of Radiology
University Hospital LMU Munich
Munich, Germany

Julian Dobranowski, MD, FRCPC, FCAR
Professor and Chair of Radiology
Faculty of Health Sciences
McMaster University
Hamilton, Ontario, Canada

Ghaneh Fananapazir, MD
Professor
Department of Radiology
University of California Davis
Sacramento, California, USA

Robert Fisher, MD, FACS
Chief
Division of Transplant Surgery
Department of Surgery
Beth Israel Deaconess Medical Center
Boston, Massachusetts, USA

Marco Francone, MD, PhD
Department of Radiological, Oncological, and
   Pathological Sciences
Sapienza University/Policlinico Umberto I
Rome, Italy

Maya Galperin-Aizenberg, MD
Cardiothoracic Imaging Division
Department of Radiology
University of Pennsylvania Health System
Assistant Professor of Clinical Radiology
Perelman School of Medicine at the University of
  Pennsylvania
Philadelphia, Pennsylvania, USA

Alejandro Garces-Descovich, MD
Diagnostic Radiology Resident
Department of Radiology
ChristianaCare Health System
Newark, Delaware, USA

Shlomit Goldberg-Stein, MD
Associate Professor of Radiology
Director, Operational Improvement
Director, Musculoskeletal Intervention
Department of Radiology
Montefiore Medical Center
Bronx, New York, USA

Marta E. Heilbrun, MD
Vice Chair of Quality
Department of Radiology and Imaging Sciences
Emory University School of Medicine
Atlanta, Georgia, USA

Nicole Hindman, MD
Associate Professor
Department of Radiology and Department of Surgery
New York University School of Medicine
New York, New York, USA

Jenny K. Hoang, MBBS, MHS, MBA
Neuroradiology Faculty
Vice Chair and Medical Director
Associate Professor of Radiology
Department of Radiology and Radiological Science
Johns Hopkins University School of Medicine
Baltimore, Maryland, USA

Michael J. Hoch, MD
Assistant Professor
Department of Radiology
Pennsylvania University Hospital
Philadelphia, Pennsylvania, USA

Jeanne M. Horowitz, MD
Associate Professor of Abdominal Imaging
Department of Radiology
Feinberg School of Medicine
Northwestern University
Chicago, Illinois, USA

Eric M. Hu, MD, MPH
Diagnostic Radiologist
Department of Radiology
Intermountain Healthcare
Salt Lake City, Utah, USA

Priyanka Jha, MBBS
Associate Professor
Department of Radiology and Biomedical Imaging
University of California San Francisco
San Francisco, California, USA

Katherine Kaproth-Joslin, MD, PhD
Assistant Professor
Department of Imaging Sciences
University of Rochester
Rochester, New York, USA

Donald Kim, DO
Assistant Professor of Radiology
Department of Radiology
Northwestern University
Chicago, Illinois, USA

Rachael R. Kirkbride, MBChB
Research Fellow
Cardiothoracic Imaging Section
Department of Radiology
Beth Israel Deaconess Medical Center
Harvard Medical School
Boston, Massachusetts, USA

Seth Kligerman, MD
Associate Professor
Division Chief of Cardiothoracic Radiology
University of California, San Diego
La Jolla, California, USA

Doenja M.J. Lambregts, MD, PhD
Radiologist
Department of Radiology
The Netherlands Cancer Institute
Amsterdam, the Netherlands

Diana Litmanovich, MD, FNASCI
Chief
Cardiothoracic Imaging Section
Department of Radiology
Beth Israel Deaconess Medical Center
Associate Professor of Radiology
Harvard Medical School
Boston, Massachusetts, USA

Thomas W. Loehfelm, MD, PhD
Assistant Professor
Department of Radiology
UC Davis Medical Center
Sacramento, California, USA

David A. Lynch, MB BCh
Professor
Department of Radiology
National Jewish Health
Denver, Colorado, USA

Mark D. Mamlouk, MD
Co-Interim Neuroradiology Lead
The Permanente Medical Group
Santa Clara, California, USA
Adjunct Assistant Professor of Neuroradiology
University of California
San Francisco, California, USA

Kathryn McGillen, MD
Assistant Professor
Department of Radiology
Penn State Health
Hershey, Pennsylvania, USA

Koenraad J. Mortele, MD
Abdominal Radiologist
Boston, Massachusetts, USA

Stephanie Nougaret, MD, PhD
Attending Radiologist
MRI Director
Department of Radiology
Montpellier Cancer Institute
University of Montpellier
Montpellier, France

Paul M. Parizel, MD, PhD, FRANZCR
David Hartley Chair of Radiology
Department of Radiology
University of Western Australia (UWA) and Royal
    Perth Hospital (RPH)
Perth, Western Australia, Australia

Krupa K. Patel-Lippmann, MD
Assistant Professor
Department of Radiology and Radiologic Sciences
Vanderbilt University Medical Center
Nashville, Tennessee, USA

Milena Petranovic, MD
Radiologist
Division of Thoracic Imaging and Intervention
Department of Radiology
Massachusetts General Hospital
Boston, Massachusetts, USA

Liina Poder, MD
Professor and Director of Ultrasound
Department of Radiology and Biomedical Imaging
University of California San Francisco
San Francisco, California, USA

Jessica B. Robbins, MD
Vice Chair Faculty Development and Enrichment
Department of Radiology
University of Wisconsin School of Medicine and
    Public Health
Madison, Wisconsin, USA

Elizabeth A. Sadowski, MD
Professor and Director of Gynecologic Imaging
Departments of Radiology, Obstetrics and
    Gynecology
University of Wisconsin School of Medicine and
    Public Health
Madison, Wisconsin, USA

Hakan Sahin, MD
Assistant Professor
Department of Radiology
Renaissance School of Medicine at Stony Brook
    University
Stony Brook, New York, USA

Rodrigo Salgado, MD, PhD
Department of Radiology
Antwerp University Hospital and Holy Heart Hospital
  Lier
Belgium

Cornelia Schaefer-Prokop, MD
Department of Radiology
Meander Medical Center
Amersfoort, the Netherlands

Khoschy Schawkat, MD
Radiologist
Department of Radiology
Brigham and Women's Hospital/Dana Farber Cancer
  Institute
Boston, Massachusetts, USA

Anuradha S. Shenoy-Bhangle, MD
Fellowship Program Director
Staff Radiologist
Abdominal Imaging and Interventions
Department of Radiology
Beth Israel Deaconess Medical Centre
Harvard Medical School
Boston, Massachusetts, USA

Atul B. Shinagare, MD
Chief of Abdominal Imaging and Intervention
Department of Radiology
Brigham and Women's Hospital/Harvard University
Boston, Massachusetts, USA

Wieland H. Sommer*, MD, MPH
Professor of Radiology
Head of Oncologic Imaging
Department of Clinical Radiology
Ludwig Maximilians University
Munich, Germany

Benjamin D. Spilseth, MD, MBA
Associate Professor
Medical Director of Body Imaging
Department of Radiology
University of Minnesota
Minneapolis, Minnesota, USA

Edward J. Tanner, MD
Chief of Gynecologic Oncology
Department of Obstetrics and Gynecology
Feinberg School of Medicine
Northwestern Unviersity
Chicago, Illinois, USA

Temel Tirkes, MD, FACR
Associate Professor of Radiology and Urology
Director of Genitourinary Radiology
Department of Radiology and Imaging Sciences
Indiana University School of Medicine
Indianapolis, Indiana, USA

Parag P. Tolat, MD
Associate Professor of Radiology and Surgery
Department of Radiology
Medical College of Wisconsin
Milwaukee, Wisconsin, USA

Daniela M. Tridente, MD
Clinical Fellow
Cardiothoracic Imaging
Department of Radiology
Beth Israel Deaconess Medical Center
Harvard Medical School
Boston, Massachusetts, USA

Susan Tsai, MD
Associate Professor of Surgery
Department of Surgical Oncology
Medical College of Wisconsin
Milwaukee, Wisconsin, USA

Thijs Vande Vyvere, PhD
Researcher
Department of Radiology
University of Antwerp and Antwerp University
  Hospital
Edegem, Antwerp, Belgium

Brent D. Weinberg, MD, PhD
Assistant Professor
Department of Radiology and Imaging Sciences
Emory University
Atlanta, Georgia, USA

Jeffrey L. Weinstein, MD, FSIR
Section of Vascular and Interventional Radiology
Program Director
Vascular and Interventional Radiology Residency
    Programs
Beth Israel Deaconess Medical Center
Boston, Massachusetts, USA

Benjamin Wildman-Tobriner, MD
Assistant Professor of Radiology
Duke University Hospital
Durham, North Carolina, USA

Marta Wojewodzka, MD
Assistant
Department of Endocrine Oncology and Nuclear
    Medicine
Maria Sklodowska-Curie National Research Institute
    of Oncology
Warsaw, Poland

Carol Wu, MD
Professor
Department of Thoracic Imaging
University of Texas MD Anderson Cancer Center
Houston, Texas, USA

Xin (Cynthia) Wu, MD
Assistant Professor
Department of Radiology and Imaging Sciences
Emory University School of Medicine
Atlanta, Georgia, USA

S. Paran Yap, MD, MBA
Radiology Resident
Department of Radiology
UC Davis Medical Center
Sacramento, California, USA

Judy Yee, MD, FACR
University Chair and Professor
Department of Radiology
Albert Einstein College of Medicine
Montefiore Medical Center
New York, New York, USA

*Dr. Wieland H. Sommer is the founder of Smart Reporting GmbH, a company for structured reporting.

Section I

What Is Structured Reporting and Do We Need It?

1 What is Structured Reporting? Clarifying the Meaning

Julian Dobranowski

The purpose of radiology report is to provide information to stakeholders about clinical decision support. Organizational guidelines exist that outline the components of a good radiological report.[1,2] Qualities of optimized radiological reports include clarity, correctness, confidence, concision, completeness, consistency, communication, and consultation as well as good form and style.[3]

Despite the existence of these guidelines, issues related to the quality of radiology reports continue to exist and need to be addressed.[4]

1.1 Effective Communication and the Stakeholders

Communication is the process of transmitting information and common understanding from one person to another.[5] It has a sender of information and a receiver of information. Written communication is the use of words to exchange information. In radiology the stakeholders are all participants of the communication process.

Communication in radiology can be erroneously viewed as a one-way process between the radiologist (sender) and the referring physician (receiver), but it is a more complex phenomenon that starts with the physician who decides to refer the patient to the radiologist and ends when the interpreted information is effectively communicated to the multiple stakeholders. Effective communication requires that the transmitted content is received and understood by the stakeholders in the way it was intended.[6] We have identified over 16 stakeholders that may require the radiological report for a computed tomography (CT) examination of the thorax performed for lung cancer staging (see ► Fig. 1.1). They include referring physicians, pathologists, other radiologists, and the patients. Each requires the information to make clinical decisions that impact patient outcomes.

Recent articles highlight the lack of information leading to a quality gap in communication.[7,8] Structured reporting is an opportunity for radiology to address this quality gap by engaging multistakeholders, understanding what information is needed, and facilitating radiologists who provide this information.

1.2 What is Disease-Specific Structured Reporting?

The Merriam-Webster's Dictionary defines communication as something arranged in a definite pattern of organization.[9] Structured reporting in health care refers to a clinical report whose content is structured at one or more levels of detail.

There is variation in the definition of structured reporting used in the radiology literature. Definitions range from the use of a simple given set of subheadings to the use of discrete fields for specific diseases and fully analyzable data based on standardized radiological terminologies. Words used synonymously with structured reporting are standardized reporting, templated reporting, and proforma reporting.

From a quality perspective and for a better understanding of the current status of reporting and preparing for the future, it is convenient to look at structured reporting from levels of structure.

Building on a previously reported three-level spectrum,[10] a six-level spectrum for structured reporting (► Table 1.1) has been proposed.[11] Each level has clearly distinguishing characteristics. Levels 1–3 relate to form, whereas levels 4–6 address content and are disease specific.

Improving the quality of the radiology reports by improving completeness can be achieved at level 4. Effective communication is addressed at level 5. The quality of report data for analyses increases as the level of structure in the report increases. Level 6 is also referred to as "synoptic" reporting.

1.3 The Future

The full benefit of radiological structured reporting will be realized when level 6 (synoptic reporting) is widely achieved. Synoptic reporting is the highest level of structured reporting where the full radiological report is in discrete data field format. This level of structured reporting will allow for the standardization of the report information and for the sharing of this information between clinical information systems. It will also allow for real-time staging, advanced analytics, research, augmented peer learning, and the training of artificial intelligence algorithms.

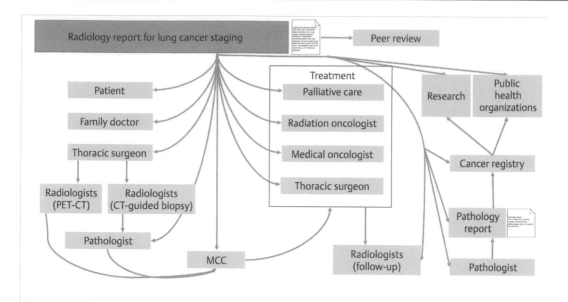

Fig. 1.1 Stakeholders requiring the radiological report. (Reproduced with permission of Dobranowski, J., Sommer W. Structured radiology reporting: addressing the communication quality gap. SN Compr. Clin. Med. 1,400 [2019]).

Table 1.1 Six levels of structured reporting[11]

Level	Attributes	Add
1	No structure No standardized elements	
2	Structure with section headers, no structured elements	Add to 1 Section headers
3	Structure with section and subsection headers, no structured elements	Add to 2 Subsection headers
4	Structure with section and subsection headers, structured elements	Add to 3 Structured elements
5	Structure with section and subsection headers, expert panel–derived structured elements	Add to 4 Expert panel, multistakeholder
6	Structure with section and subsection headers, expert panel–derived structured elements, saved in discrete data elements—synoptic	Add to 5 Discrete fields, data mining enabled

References

[1] American College of Radiology (2008). ACR practice guideline for the communication of diagnostic imaging findings. https://www.acr.org/-/media/ACR/Files/Practice-Parameters/CommunicationDiag.pdf. Accessed March 11, 2019

[2] European Society of Radiology (ESR), Guidelines from the European Society of Radiology (ESR). Good practice for radiological reporting. Insights Imaging. 2011; 2(2):93–96

[3] Flanders AE, Lakhani P. Radiology reporting and communications: a look forward. Neuroimaging Clin N Am. 2012; 22(3):477–496

[4] Waite S, Scott J, Gale B, Fuchs T, Kolla S, Reede D. Interpretive error in radiology. AJR Am J Roentgenol. 2017; 208(4):739–749

[5] Keyton J. Communication and organizational culture: a key to understanding work experience. 2nd ed. Thousand Oaks, CA: Sage; 2010

[6] Stewart MA. Effective physician-patient communication and health outcomes: a review. CMAJ. 1995; 152(9):1423–1433

[7] Brook OR, Brook A, Vollmer CM, Kent TS, Sanchez N, Pedrosa I. Structured reporting of multiphasic CT for pancreatic cancer: potential effect on staging and surgical planning. Radiology. 2015; 274(2):464–472

[8] Nörenberg D, Sommer WH, Thasler W, et al. Structured reporting of rectal magnetic resonance imaging in suspected primary rectal cancer: potential benefits for surgical planning and interdisciplinary communication. Invest Radiol. 2017; 52(4):232–239

[9] "Structure." Merriam-Webster.com. Merriam-Webster Incorporated. https://www.merriam-webster.com/dictionary/communication. Accessed March 11, 2019

[10] Weiss DL, Langlotz CP. Structured reporting: patient care enhancement or productivity nightmare? Radiology. 2008; 249(3):739–747

[11] Dobranowski, J., Sommer W. Structured radiology reporting: addressing the communication quality gap. SN Compr. Clin. Med. 1, 397–407 (2019). https://doi.org/10.1007/s42399-019-00066-5

2 Pros and Cons of Structured Reporting

Charlotte Y. Chung, Hernan R. Bello, and Marta E. Heilbrun

2.1 Introduction

As mentioned in the first chapter, the radiology report is the vehicle by which an individual radiologist communicates his or her interpretation of an imaging study with referring providers and patients. For decades, prose-style reporting has been used, reflecting a radiologist's expertise in the art and practice of medicine. In the past several years, structured and templated reporting has emerged as an alternative. The advocates of this style believe that it improves ease and speed of comprehension in an overburdened clinical environment. There are different levels of structured reporting, ranging from simple subheadings to fully synoptic reports. Currently, up to 90% of academic radiology practices in the United States have implemented some form of structured reporting, with 50% having done so for over half of their total volume.[1] However, the radiology community has yet to fully embrace this practice, with concerns related to the perceived rigidity, potential for errors, and fear of commoditization limiting radiologists' widespread adoption and satisfaction of structured and templated reporting.[1,2,3]

The ultimate goal of a radiologist is to combine image information and clinical acumen to facilitate the care of their patients. This is realized by the successful communication of their interpretations to their referring providers and patients. The field of radiology needs to find the correct balance between efficiently producing a product that provides the most value to the customers while at the same time preserving the autonomy and supporting the expertise of the radiologist. Understanding the advantages and disadvantages of structured reporting is paramount.

2.2 Pros of Structured Reporting

2.2.1 Preference

- There is a preference for structured reports in the majority of referring providers[1,4,5,6] because the uniform organization and consistent vocabulary improve readability and reduce ambiguity, particularly for actionable information and recommendations.[7]

2.2.2 Efficiency and Accuracy

- Efficiency is improved, both for the interpreting radiologist (decreased dictation and report turnaround time)[8] and for the referring provider (quicker comprehension and consumption).[9]
- The use of checklists, prepopulated fields, and/or pick-lists can reduce diagnostic errors from "satisfaction of search"[10] and/or failure to report incidental findings,[11,12] and decrease the incidence of grammatical and nongrammatical voice recognition errors.[13]

2.2.3 Quality Metric Tracking and Data Mining

- Compliance to radiology and external guidelines/mandates,[14] including practice guidelines that direct management recommendations (e.g., Fleischner Society pulmonary nodule guidelines and the American College of Radiology Reporting and Data Systems[15,16]) and documentation requirements to ensure reimbursements/financial incentives or avoid penalties (under the Medicare Merit-based Incentive Payment System),[17] is facilitated.
- Consistent use of terminologies based on standardized reporting language (e.g., RadLex) allows more effective analysis and tracking (potentially utilizing natural language processing) for auditing,[18] data mining for research,[19,20] clinical decision support, and quality improvement.

2.2.4 Ease of Adoption

- Disciplines with limited anatomy and/or restricted diseases, or a large proportion of negative/screening studies, such as breast and cardiac imaging, readily adopted this style.[21,22]
- Structured templates, especially when contextual (e.g., disease-specific),[23,24] provide content tailored to the diagnosis/indication, ensuring relevance and completeness (inclusion of all pertinent positives and negatives) of report findings, particularly for less frequently encountered conditions.[25,26,27]
- Availability of existing resources on standardized language such as RadLex,[28] structured report libraries,[29] and resources provided by specific

radiological subspecialty societies (e.g., Society of Interventional Radiology and Society for Abdominal Radiology) leverages the expertise of our profession, potentially disseminating improved care.

2.2.5 Integration with New Technologies

- Offers a framework for incorporating emerging reporting solutions, such as decision support for radiologist report recommendations[30] and multimedia-enhanced reports,[31] to further enhance evidence-based medicine and value of the radiology report.[9]

2.2.6 Education

- Structured templates can be leveraged as a training tool for radiology residents to learn the art of framing a radiology report, while forcing careful examination of all structures before dictating every single anatomic structure as "normal."[17,32]

2.3 Cons of Structured Reporting

2.3.1 Risk of Commoditization

- Hand-crafted prose reports reflect a radiologist's individuality and art of radiology reporting. Uniform reporting takes away personal connection with referring providers and may commoditize our specialty.[17,33]

2.3.2 Concern for Errors

- Unclear benefits for improving accuracy of interpretation[34,35] and/or comprehension of radiology reports.[36]
- Potentially increased errors if prepopulated "normal" fields were inappropriately kept in the template.[1,37]
- Increased interaction with the reporting system and focus on template adherence could distract from image interpretation, disrupt existing search pattern and cognitive reasoning, ultimately reducing diagnostic accuracy and/or efficiency.[7,33]

2.3.3 Efficiency

- Customization of structured templates is needed to meet the needs of various referring physicians

or to tailor structured templates to particular disease conditions, resulting in slower report production.
- Prose-form dictation style is inherently flexible and customizable, and thus particularly preferred among older radiologists.[4,33,38]
- Significant decrease in productivity negatively impacts radiology workflow during initial implementation[7,17] due to a steep learning curve, time and effort to develop and maintain report templates, and variable existing resources for overcoming institutional resistance.

2.3.4 Unnatural Reporting and Oversimplification

- Rigid structure of the report template leads to the issues of overfragmentation and overcompleteness.[2]
  - Complex multisystem disease process with findings unnaturally divided over several sections is difficult and more time-consuming to describe/dictate and equally hard to comprehend.
  - Forced inclusion of unnecessary or irrelevant information in a predetermined order can mask important information, decreasing coherence and usefulness of the report.[7,17,39]
- Oversimplification of the radiology report, particularly for sophisticated or complex studies, may create the illusion that the interpreting radiologist is neither knowledgeable nor thorough, causing distrust and dissatisfaction among referring providers.[37,40]

2.3.5 Education

- Concern with possible negative impact on radiology resident education by allowing cursory viewing of exams,[32] particularly hindering learning with describing pathology, synthesizing, and/or interpreting findings.[1]

In conclusion, while there are valid arguments against structured and templated reporting, we believe the benefits outweigh these arguments. With the emergence of new reporting technologies, contextual and disease-specific templates, learning in electronic environments, and in anticipation of future incorporation of artificial intelligence in the radiologist's work environment, a reporting system that is unorganized will be insufficient to deliver the value that the radiologist brings to the patient experience.

References

[1] Powell DK, Silberzweig JE. State of structured reporting in radiology: a survey. Acad Radiol. 2015; 22(2):226–233

[2] Faggioni L, Coppola F, Ferrari R, Neri E, Regge D. Usage of structured reporting in radiological practice: results from an Italian online survey. Eur Radiol. 2017; 27(5):1934–1943

[3] Bosmans JML, Weyler JJ, De Schepper AM, Parizel PM. The radiology report as seen by radiologists and referring clinicians: results of the COVER and ROVER surveys. Radiology. 2011; 259(1):184–195

[4] Schwartz LH, Panicek DM, Berk AR, Li Y, Hricak H. Improving communication of diagnostic radiology findings through structured reporting. Radiology. 2011; 260(1):174–181

[5] Lather JD, Che Z, Saltzman B, Bieszczad J. Structured reporting in the academic setting: what the referring clinician wants. J Am Coll Radiol. 2018; 15(5):772–775

[6] Dickerson E, Davenport MS, Syed F, et al. Michigan Radiology Quality Collaborative. Effect of template reporting of brain MRIs for multiple sclerosis on report thoroughness and neurologist-rated quality: results of a prospective quality improvement project. J Am Coll Radiol. 2017; 14 (3):371–379.e1

[7] Cramer JA, Eisenmenger LB, Pierson NS, Dhatt HS, Heilbrun ME. Structured and templated reporting: an overview. Appl Radiol. 2014; 43(8):18–21. Accessed February 11, 2019

[8] Jain B, Bhagwat K, Shashikiran R, et al. Structured reporting of facial skeletal trauma CT scan as a tool to reduce report turnaround time (TAT). 2017. doi:10.1594/ecr2017/B-0103

[9] Eberhardt SC, Heilbrun ME. Radiology report value equation. Radiographics. 2018; 38(6):1888–1896

[10] Lin E, Powell DK, Kagetsu NJ. Efficacy of a checklist-style structured radiology reporting template in reducing resident misses on cervical spine computed tomography examinations. J Digit Imaging. 2014; 27(5):588–593

[11] Quattrocchi CC, Giona A, Di Martino AC, et al. Extra-spinal incidental findings at lumbar spine MRI in the general population: a large cohort study. Insights Imaging. 2013; 4 (3):301–308

[12] Semaan HB, Bieszczad JE, Obri T, et al. Incidental extraspinal findings at lumbar spine magnetic resonance imaging: a retrospective study. Spine. 2015; 40(18):1436–1443

[13] Hawkins CM, Hall S, Zhang B, Towbin AJ. Creation and implementation of department-wide structured reports: an analysis of the impact on error rate in radiology reports. J Digit Imaging. 2014; 27(5):581–587

[14] Kahn CE, Jr, Heilbrun ME, Applegate KE. From guidelines to practice: how reporting templates promote the use of radiology practice guidelines. J Am Coll Radiol. 2013; 10 (4):268–273

[15] MacMahon H, Naidich DP, Goo JM, et al. Guidelines for management of incidental pulmonary nodules detected on CT images: from the Fleischner Society 2017. Radiology. 2017; 284(1):228–243

[16] American College of Radiology. Reporting and data systems. https://www.acr.org/Clinical-Resources/Reporting-and-Data-Systems. Accessed February 13, 2019

[17] Ganeshan D, Duong PT, Probyn L, et al. Structured reporting in radiology. Acad Radiol. 2018; 25(1):66–73

[18] Burnside ES, Sickles EA, Bassett LW, et al. The ACR BI-RADS experience: learning from history. J Am Coll Radiol. 2009; 6 (12):851–860

[19] Orel SG, Kay N, Reynolds C, Sullivan DC. BI-RADS categorization as a predictor of malignancy. Radiology. 1999; 211 (3):845–850

[20] Liberman L, Abramson AF, Squires FB, Glassman JR, Morris EA, Dershaw DD. The breast imaging reporting and data system: positive predictive value of mammographic features and final assessment categories. AJR Am J Roentgenol. 1998; 171(1):35–40

[21] D'Orsi C, Sickles E, Mendelson E, Morris E. ACR BI-RADS® Atlas, Breast Imaging Reporting and Data System. Reston, VA: American College of Radiology; 2013. https://scholar.google. com/scholar_lookup?title=ACR%20BI-RADS%20atlas%3A% 20breast%20imaging%20reporting%20and%20data%20 system&publication_year=2013&author=American%20Col-lege%20of%20Radiology. Accessed February 13, 2019

[22] Stillman AE, Rubin GD, Teague SD, White RD, Woodard PK, Larson PA. Structured reporting: coronary CT angiography: a white paper from the American College of Radiology and the North American Society for Cardiovascular Imaging. J Am Coll Radiol. 2008; 5(7):796–800

[23] RSNA 2017: Contextual radiology reporting templates: Structured Reporting 2.0? https://appliedradiology.com/articles/ rsna-2017-contextual-radiology-reporting-templates-structured-reporting-2-0. Accessed February 13, 2019

[24] Mamlouk MD, Chang PC, Saket RR. Contextual radiology reporting: a new approach to neuroradiology structured templates. AJNR Am J Neuroradiol. 2018; 39(8):1406–1414

[25] Brook OR, Brook A, Vollmer CM, Kent TS, Sanchez N, Pedrosa I. Structured reporting of multiphasic CT for pancreatic cancer: potential effect on staging and surgical planning. Radiology. 2015; 274(2):464–472

[26] Sahni VA, Silveira PC, Sainani NI, Khorasani R. Impact of a structured report template on the quality of MRI reports for rectal cancer staging. AJR Am J Roentgenol. 2015; 205 (3):584–588

[27] Marcovici PA, Taylor GA. Journal club: structured radiology reports are more complete and more effective than unstructured reports. AJR Am J Roentgenol. 2014; 203(6):1265–1271

[28] RSNA. RadLex. Radiological Society of North America. http:// radlex.org/. Accessed February 13, 2019

[29] RSNA. RadReport. http://radreport.org/. Accessed February 13, 2019

[30] Boland GWL, Thrall JH, Gazelle GS, et al. Decision support for radiologist report recommendations. J Am Coll Radiol. 2011; 8(12):819–823

[31] Folio LR, Machado LB, Dwyer AJ. Multimedia-enhanced radiology reports: concept, components, and challenges. Radiographics. 2018; 38(2):462–482

[32] Bosmans JML, Peremans L, Menni M, De Schepper AM, Duyck PO, Parizel PM. Structured reporting: if, why, when, how-and at what expense? Results of a focus group meeting of radiology professionals from eight countries. Insights Imaging. 2012; 3(3):295–302

[33] Weiss DL, Langlotz CP. Structured reporting: patient care enhancement or productivity nightmare? Radiology. 2008; 249(3):739–747

[34] Johnson AJ, Chen MYM, Swan JS, Applegate KE, Littenberg B. Cohort study of structured reporting compared with conventional dictation. Radiology. 2009; 253(1):74–80

[35] Hawkins CM, Hall S, Hardin J, Salisbury S, Towbin AJ. Prepopulated radiology report templates: a prospective analysis of error rate and turnaround time. J Digit Imaging. 2012; 25(4):504–511

[36] Sistrom CL, Honeyman-Buck J. Free text versus structured format: information transfer efficiency of radiology reports. AJR Am J Roentgenol. 2005; 185(3):804–812

[37] Reinus WR. Economics of radiology report editing using voice recognition technology. J Am Coll Radiol. 2007; 4 (12):890–894

[38] Gunderman RB, McNeive LR. Is structured reporting the answer? Radiology. 2014; 273(1):7–9

[39] Ash JS, Berg M, Coiera E. Some unintended consequences of information technology in health care: the nature of patient care information system-related errors. J Am Med Inform Assoc. 2004; 11(2):104–112

[40] Boland GW, Duszak R, Jr. Structured reporting and communication. J Am Coll Radiol. 2015; 12 12 Pt A:1286–1288

3 Change Management—How to Implement Structured Reporting

Shlomit Goldberg-Stein and Victoria Chernyak

3.1 Introduction

The major objective of the radiology report is to provide accurate, timely, and actionable information to the referring provider. Traditional free-text reporting not only provides a high degree of radiologist autonomy, but also allows for a great deal of variability, nonstandard language, and potential ambiguity. Structured reporting has become increasingly accepted as the preferred alternative to traditional prose reporting,[1,2,3] with a growing body of literature demonstrating decreased reporting errors, superiority in the quality and comprehensiveness of reporting,[1,2,3,4] and greater adherence to accepted national guidelines.[5,6,7]

Despite many known advantages, adoption of standardized structured reporting in practice may be hindered by the need for dedicated time and resources to develop and refine templates, technical challenges, and adaptive challenges. Adaptive challenges relate to the consensus building efforts and change management techniques required to overcome resistance by radiologists to accept this major change in reporting. This is arguably the greatest hurdle to overcome in the introduction of structured radiology reporting to a group of radiologists. As mentioned in the previous chapter, besides many pros, there are also cons of structured reporting. Among those reported in the previous chapter, the adaptive challenge stems from the following legitimate concerns that radiologists may express regarding the change to structured reporting:

- Loss of freedom and autonomy.
- Altering search patterns to conform to the template, potentially resulting in interpretive error.
- Inadvertent retention of prepopulated normal statements in reports.
- Difficulty in cases where findings do not fit neatly into one section/header.

Despite the above challenges, change can be implemented successfully if strategically planned. In his seminal work entitled "Leading Change," John P. Kotter, Professor Emeritus of Leadership at the Harvard Business School, provides an eight-stage process for leaders to overcome resistance and create change.[8] Kotter's eight-stage change model aligns with another change model by Kurt Lewin

which emphasizes the need to the hardwire change that is introduced, to guarantee long-term success and prevent reversion to an earlier state of behavior.[9] Taking the wisdom of these change models together, consider the following steps in approaching the challenge of overhauling reporting (▶ Table 3.1):

- *Unfreeze*: Gently defrost the status quo, in Kotter's steps 1–4.
- *Change*: Introduce innovation, in Kotter's steps 5–7.
- *Refreeze*: Ensure the change will last, in Kotter's step 8.

In this chapter, we incorporate these concepts into a road map of how to successfully implement structured reporting in your organization, with the focus on a practical methodology that can address radiologists' fears of change. Specifically, we apply Kotter's and Lewin's models of change to the leadership challenge of how to transform radiology reporting practice within an organization.

3.2 How to Implement Structured Reporting

3.2.1 Unfreeze

In this phase, leadership is required to create a platform for change, to build a team, and to

Table 3.1 Models of change management

Kotter's eight-stage process of creating major change	Kurt Lewin's three-step change model
1. Establishing a sense of urgency	Unfreeze
2. Creating the guiding coalition	
3. Developing a vision and strategy	
4. Communicating the change vision	
5. Empowering broad-based action	Change
6. Generating short-term wins	
7. Consolidating gains and producing more change	
8. Anchoring new approaches in the culture	Freeze

Source: Adapted with permission from Kotter JP 2007.[8]

develop and then articulate a vision and strategy for reporting overhaul. Consensus building efforts in this phase are critical for the overall success of the project. The steps to take are as follows:

- *Obtain leadership support, and form a core team*: There is precedent for success with early support of the practice leadership or the Department Chair.[3] The core structured reporting team typically includes one to two project leads, who might be leaders in informatics and/or quality improvement, and ideally one administrator.
- *Prepare*: Project leads should begin by briefly reviewing relevant current literature on structured reporting and become knowledgeable about benefits and potential challenges of structured reporting.
- *Create urgency*: Share knowledge with faculty/staff and trainees in formal and informal forums, and present concepts at staff meetings, quality assurance sessions, divisional meetings, and in local conversations. This is the first step in beginning to loosen, or defrost, the status quo. In order to drive change, an urgent need for change is required. Without urgency, the status quo will remain the most convenient option, and radiologists will prefer to continue in the traditional reporting paradigm. In order to convey an urgent need for change, it is important to articulate the benefits of structured reporting for the patient and for the care team. *The ultimate argument for structured reporting is that it places the patient squarely at the center and furthers patient-centered care by consistently providing clear and actionable information to the care team.* Sharing published improvement data from other institutions may be helpful.[5,6,7]
- *Acknowledge a new balance*: The need to balance personal autonomy and expert opinion with standardization lies at the heart of structured reporting initiatives. Although uniform reporting of normal findings is of critical importance (i.e., language for a normal exam used by any given radiologist should match language for a normal exam used by other radiologists in the team, so there is no need for a referring care team to "interpret" the relative normalcy of any given exam report), radiologists should not be overlimited in their descriptions of abnormal findings, or in the impression section of the report, except where defined lexicon or grading/staging system (i.e., Radiology Reporting and Data Systems) is required. Preservation of autonomy in those areas is an important balancing component. In addition, be sure to

acknowledge that although some degree of radiologist freedom and autonomy is surrendered with structured reporting, this loss is outweighed by the positive effects of standardization, consistency, comparability, and adherence to national guidelines.

- *Form subspecialty teams*: A dedicated committee or team is required for template development. Teams are typically divided by specialty, and four to six teams may be required, with one team lead for each. Teams should include subspecialty leaders, and also representatives from all sites of multisite practices. Interdepartmental collaboration with nonradiologist referring physicians is critical for reports to adhere to local practice expectations; stakeholders are listed for each template in the chapters that follow, and should be included on subspecialty teams. For academic departments, residents might be included. They are often technologically savvy, and are responsible for drafting a large proportion of department reports. In addition, previous efforts have reported high levels of early template adherence by trainees.[3]
- *Develop and communicate your vision and strategy*: Project leads must develop and then share (overcommunicate!) the proposed process for structured reporting implementation. The vision should include both the technical approach and timeline (suggested technical steps are outlined in ▶ Table 3.2) and also a clear strategy for engagement and communication. Project leads must be available and responsive to needs, concerns, and fears in order to drive forward decision making in the next phase.[4]

3.2.2 Change

In this phase, report templates are created, vetted, and undergo iterative improvements and final approval. Momentum builds, and reporting overhaul takes place. For consensus building, consider the following:

- *Scope the project*: Your choice of how to scope the initial phases of the project (i.e., first batch of templates) will depend on the degree of early support anticipated from various subspecialty leaders in your department or practice. Options include: (1) begin with one modality (computed tomography [CT], magnetic resonance [MR], ultrasound [US], or X-rays); (2) begin with one subspecialty and progress through template development by team (e.g., abdominal, chest,

Table 3.2 Technical strategy: steps of template creation and multistep refinement

Step	Action
1. Template drafting	1. Subspecialty team member drafts a template with the guidance of relevant stakeholders (i.e., radiologists and referring physicians). See Chapter 4 "How to Build a Template." 2. Project leads check for use of a departmental standard header, data merge fields with patient and exam information, and ensure use of clear and grammatically correct language. Standard criteria may be developed and required of every template. Pick-list options and text fields are optimized to provide selectable language for common abnormalities and variants.
2. Template trials: iterative cycles of improvement	1. Communicate clearly the beginning of a new template trial. 2. Establish a defined mechanism for template feedback; a simple email process or survey may suffice. 3. Set the template to autopopulate in the dictation software with the launch of that exam within picture archiving and communication system (PACS) for all trialing radiologists. Input from information technology (IT) staff may be required for assistance with this and subsequent steps. 4. Define and communicate the length of template trial (e.g., 2 weeks). 5. Solicit template feedback through the established mechanism. 6. Compile and distribute feedback anonymously; establish sessions for discussion and voting if required. 7. Multiple rounds of trialing will often be required. The first round may be limited to high frequency readers only, or specialty leads, with subsequent rounds open to a wider group. 8. Project leads should obtain approval from billing/compliance team, provide final grammar edits, and standardize fields and pick-list options.
3. Template finalization	1. Finalized template autolaunches for all radiologists by default. 2. Finalized templates remain open to further improvements; feedback at any time is encouraged.

musculoskeletal); (3) begin with the most common exams first, and focus on less frequently performed exams later. For example, one institution began with the commonest 10 to 15 cross-sectional exams (CT/MR/US) for each subspecialty; note that this approach requires coordination with multiple subspecialty teams at the outset.[3] Another strategy that is relevant to any of the above options is to start broad, focusing more narrowly later, in order to obtain early wins; a previous report of successful implementation began with organ-system templates (e.g., abdominopelvic CT) and later developed disease-specific reports (e.g., pancreatic adenocarcinoma staging template).[2]

- *Creating templates*: Avoid the urge to directly adopt structured templates from national organizations or the chapters that follow. Consider instead using available templates as a starting point for template drafting. The reasons for this are twofold. First, there is a need to address and incorporate local standards into your templates. Second, direct staff radiologist involvement in template creation will directly counteract feelings of lost autonomy and will engage radiologists in the initiative. Similarly, as stated above, involvement of referring physicians is critical in implementing reports that will be acceptable and appreciated by the care team. This approach will contribute to willing adoption of structured reporting in your organization.

- *Iterative cycles of improvement*: Use multiple cycles of template improvement in order to maximize radiologist engagement. The process starts with template drafting, which includes input from all stakeholders (radiologists and nonradiologists). This is followed by cycles of trialing, feedback, voting, and template improvement. Iterative cycles should precede any final approval. All feedback must be respected and carefully considered, even if suggested changes are not ultimately incorporated. Most importantly, "finalized" templates should always remain open to reconsideration and further improvement.

- *Template feedback*: Establish a clear process for submission of suggestions to improve or edit report templates. If there is a clear process in place, and communication is made simple, everyone has ample opportunity to be involved. Having this process established and communicated to the involved staff is critical in engaging all radiologists. If there is a fair and predictable process for template refinement, radiologists are more likely to trust and appreciate the authenticity of the effort, and accept the change.

- *Be flexible where possible*: Flexibility restores a sense of control and autonomy, and promotes buy-in from radiologists. Some opportunities for flexibility include:
  - Adherence: Define the goal of adherence to the use of templates at <100% (perhaps 90% or 95%) to allow for exceptions. This counteracts fear of difficulties using structured reporting in cases where findings do not fit neatly into one section/header.[1,2,3,4] Also encourage combining headers and sections where required by the imaged pathology.[3]
  - Normal template: Consider allowing each team to determine whether templates will include normal statements populated by default versus containing blank fields by default; if the latter approach is chosen, normal statements can be easily populated through the use of pick-list options. This flexibility provides some leeway in discussions regarding both the fear of erroneously retained normal statements and the fear of disrupted search patterns.
  - Insist on consistency: Close familiarity with templates creates predictability and ease of use, and increases the likelihood of acceptance and widespread adoption of structured reporting. For instance, every abdominopelvic CT should have identical format, order, and pick-list options as its skeleton structure and content. Disease-specific abdominal CT templates will include additional or more lengthy sections within the standard template, which is otherwise identical to the skeleton template.[1,2,3,4] In addition, similar or identical language should be applied to describe the same anatomy in different reports; for example, if a single template is used for a combined CT head-and-neck exam, the same language and structure should be found in the CT head and CT neck individual report templates.
  - Provide incentives: Some practices have successfully used small financial incentives[1] and others have not.[3] This may be considered, depending on culture and work environment.

3.2.3 Freeze

In this phase, adherence to the use of reporting templates becomes normative and the new practice becomes ingrained in the workflow of radiologists. To be successful in this phase:

- *Make change easier*: Be fastidious that all templates are linked to their exam codes, such that automatic launching of the appropriate template occurs consistently. This is critical to sustained adherence to the use of structured report templates. Any added steps requiring searching the template library for the correct template will discourage their consistent use. With automatic launching, structured reporting becomes the new default. Deviating from template use requires additional time and effort on the part of the radiologist, and is thus less likely to occur. To achieve this, the creation of new exam codes may be required, to match unique templates.

- *Share data*: Report audits and sharing of template use-data are critical for long-term success. If there are areas where lower rates of adherence are identified (e.g., pelvic US), it is imperative to identify the underlying causes and address them quickly.

- *Outliers*: Approach any dissenting radiologist not adhering to the use of templates to privately and respectfully discuss barriers to adoption. Recommend the use of the established process for submission of suggestions to improve the report templates. An overtly respectful and inclusive approach can engage outlier radiologists and encourage compliance.

3.3 Conclusion

Kotter's and Lewin's models of change can be applied to overcome the fear of change and formulate a blueprint for successful implementation of structured reporting in your organization.

References

[1] Larson DB, Towbin AJ, Pryor RM, Donnelly LF. Improving consistency in radiology reporting through the use of department-wide standardized structured reporting. Radiology. 2013; 267(1):240–250

[2] Herts BR, Gandhi NS, Schneider E, et al. How we do it: creating consistent structure and content in abdominal radiology report templates. AJR Am J Roentgenol. 2019; 212 (3):490–496

[3] Goldberg-Stein S, Walter WR, Amis ES, Jr, Scheinfeld MH. Implementing a structured reporting initiative using a

collaborative multistep approach. Curr Probl Diagn Radiol. 2017; 46(4):295–299

[4] Larson DB. Strategies for implementing a standardized structured radiology reporting program. Radiographics. 2018; 38(6):1705–1716

[5] Kahn CE, Jr, Heilbrun ME, Applegate KE. From guidelines to practice: how reporting templates promote the use of radiology practice guidelines. J Am Coll Radiol. 2013; 10 (4):268–273

[6] Chernyak V, Fowler KJ, Kamaya A, et al. Liver Imaging Reporting and Data System (LI-RADS) Version 2018: imaging of hepatocellular carcinoma in at-risk patients. Radiology. 2018; 289(3):816–830

[7] Al-Hawary MM, Francis IR, Chari ST, et al. Pancreatic ductal adenocarcinoma radiology reporting template: consensus statement of the Society of Abdominal Radiology and the American Pancreatic Association. Radiology. 2014; 270 (1):248–260

[8] Kotter JP. Leading change: Why transformation efforts fail. Harvard Business Review. 2007 [online]. Available at: https://hbr.org/2007/01/leading-change-why-transformation-efforts-fail

[9] Lewin K. Frontiers in group dynamics: concept, method and reality in social science; social equilibria and social change. Hum Relat. 1947; 1(1):5–41

4 How to Build a Template

Thomas J.T. Anderson

4.1 The Anatomy of a Template

Templates are constructed from several core elements, each of which is typically surrounded by a special kind of bracket—such as [ ] or { }. The brackets allow the dictation software to identify and navigate between these "fields" using the buttons on a dictaphone, but the brackets themselves are not included in the text of the published report. By incorporating some or all of these different elements in series, a block of structured text can be created to address almost any scenario.

- *Blank fields*: Brackets with no internal content that are used for free text dictation. Empty brackets allow the dictation software to easily navigate to a specific place in the report, permitting the author to use free text to describe unanticipated findings or to provide a number or description in the appropriate place within a larger block of structured text.
- *Plain text*: Similar to text that would be typed or dictated into a report. Plain text makes up the majority of most blocks of structured text, using standardized language that is generic enough to be applied to many normal studies. When plain text does not need to be modified by the report author, the enclosing brackets are discouraged as they unnecessarily slow down report navigation.
- *Tokens*: Fields that provide examination-specific information such as the exact name of the examination or the clinical history. Tokens are unique, in that they require communication with an outside program to deliver the correct information. Fields of this kind are likely to be put to more frequent use in the future as newer software in imaging equipment will allow more information to be sent directly to the report, such as measurements acquired during an ultrasound examination or the specific MRI sequences that were obtained. Third-party software that analyzes radiology images could also communicate directly with the dictation software or the radiology information system (RIS) via tokens to automatically insert results.
- *Pick-lists:* Fields where one of several standard blocks of text can be chosen for incorporation into the report. Dictation software will display the available options to the report author when the pick-list field is highlighted so the appropriate option can be chosen. Many options of any length can be included in the pick-list, but often only the first portion of the text is easily readable, so it is important to make each option clear for the report author at the very beginning of the text. A default option can be included in the pick-list so that no action is needed if the default is appropriate. However, the use of a default option may lead to the accidental inclusion of incorrect or even conflicting statements if the report is not proofread carefully. These errors are not trivial and result in confusion on the part of the referring clinician and patient, who may wonder if the images were thoroughly examined or if the report was assigned to the wrong patient.

4.2 Planning a Template

Blocks of structured text can be divided into two primary types: general templates that include the entire structure and content of a full radiology report; and disease-specific templates that characterize or quantify a specific finding. The former is typically chosen or inserted at the initiation of the dictation, ideally automatically, while the latter is inserted anywhere in the report during the process of interpretation. A hybrid approach, where the full template automatically includes disease-specific language in the appropriate section(s), is useful for common diseases, especially when they impact multiple organ systems; however, it requires the creation and maintenance of more templates, and ensuring consistency of structure and language between similar templates can become difficult. Using a much smaller number of more general templates, and then inserting the disease-specific structured text as needed, makes template updating much easier and also improves the success rate of the dictation software in selecting the proper template at the start of dictation.

4.3 Creating a New Template

Building a new template begins within your chosen dictation software. All commercially available dictation software includes some method of creating, editing, and managing structured text, which may be referred to as "autotext," "macro," or "template," depending on the software. When creating a new block of structured text, the first step is to give it a name. This name is typically displayed in a long list of available templates that can be inserted, and choosing a succinct but unambiguous name is very important and more difficult than it may seem. These lists of available templates are often sorted alphabetically, so adhering to a consistent naming schema will make the process of finding the correct template substantially easier. Beginning the name with an appropriate general prefix and getting progressively more specific will help keep the lists of templates more organized.

In addition to naming a new template, each new template must be linked to certain types of examinations so that the dictation software knows when to offer that template as an option based on the specific type of study that is being reported. This is typically done by associating the template with a modality and one or more body parts, or with specific procedure codes in the RIS. Other attributes such as patient sex and age can be assigned as well in some software. When the report for a study is first created, the dictation system will search its database for all templates that match the study's parameters and display a list of the appropriate templates. Comprehensive general templates should be associated with as few examination types as possible to make the selection process as specific as possible, helping to ensure the proper template is loaded automatically, while disease-specific templates should be associated with as many examination types as possible to ensure they are available whenever the finding is made. A general template for a chest CT, for example, should not be associated with the cervical spine; however, a template for recommending follow up of pulmonary nodules should be associated not only with the chest, but also with the cervical spine and the abdomen as these examinations often include portions of the lung.

4.4 Comprehensive Templates

Creating a comprehensive template should begin by entering general section headings such as "Examination," "Indication," "Technique," "Comparison," "Findings," "Impression," "Recommendations," and/or "Communication." Consistent formatting with a large, bold font is important to make these section headings stand out for easy readability for both the report author and the report audience, while subsection headings should be consecutively smaller and less conspicuous, using similar formatting for headings at similar levels in the hierarchy.

- *Examination and indication*: Typically automatically imported through the use of tokens, while the remaining sections will need to be entered manually.
- *Technique*: A combination of plain text, pick-lists, and tokens. If there are several different ways to perform the type of study at hand, pick-lists can be used to choose between them, either choosing a few words here and there, such as "{with/without}," or the pick-list options can each include a comprehensive technique section. Similar to template naming, pick-list options may not display long blocks of text very well and starting each option with a clear label is recommended.
- *Comparison*: More variable with a blank field, a field that just says "{None.}", or a pick-list with multiple options followed by a blank field: "{None./Prior CTs dated } { }" all being reasonable approaches.
- *Findings*: General templates should utilize an organ- or systems-based approach. A plain text section heading for each organ or system can be followed either by bracketed plain text using standardized language that describes normal findings for that section, or a pick-list with options describing each of the most common findings for that section. Pick-lists should be used wherever possible with comprehensive options covering common scenarios in each field. This approach allows a report to be rapidly constructed by navigating through each field in order and choosing the appropriate option from the pick-list. Blank fields can be used to easily add additional findings to the end of a section without overwriting the existing text, or to insert a number or descriptor into a larger block of plain text.
- *Impression*: This field is the most likely to change during the course of interpretation, and several approaches are reasonable, including a blank field, a numbered list beginning with a blank field, or simply "Normal."

4.5 Disease-Specific Templates

Disease-specific structured text, examples of which will be provided throughout the rest of this book, can be incorporated directly into the more general templates described above. Depending on the length and complexity of the description, it may be useful to include section headings within the template. This information is often granular and each field is best placed on its own line, in the form of a plain text label followed by a pick-list or a blank field for the report author to enter the appropriate information. Pick-lists should be used whenever possible to help standardize reporting language.

4.6 Pearls

- Keep plain text language broad enough to encompass numerous common scenarios without requiring substantial editing.
- Use brackets around any text that may need to be changed during the course of interpretation, and avoid brackets around text that never changes.

- Include identifying information at the beginning of long pick-list options and at the end of template names.
- Pay meticulous attention to detail. Small typos will be incorporated into many reports if not detected and corrected.
- Consistency is key, and if multiple closely related general templates include the same anatomy, the descriptions should be kept the same across all templates.
- Pick-lists with default options improve efficiency of report generation but may cause incorrect or conflicting information to be included in the report and careful proofreading remains important.
- Seek feedback on templates from radiologists and referring clinicians alike to ensure that typos are corrected, missing information is added, and clarity and efficiency are improved.

Section II

Structured Reports in Cancer Imaging

Editor: Wieland H. Sommer

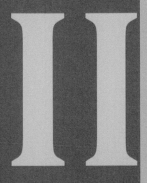

II

5 Lymphoma Staging PET-CT

Lukas Abraszek and Marta Wojewodzka

5.1 Template

Lymph nodes:
Lymphadenopathy: [yes/no]
  If yes: **present on both sides of the diaphragm:** [yes/no]
Affected regions: [Waldeyer's ring/preauricular/cervical/supraclavicular/infraclavicular/hilar/mediastinal/axillary/mesenteric/retroperitoneal/common iliac/external iliac/internal iliac/inguinal/femoral];
Side: [right/left]
Index lesion specification: (▶ Table 5.1)
Spleen:
Splenomegaly: [yes/no]
  If yes: **spleen size:** [ ] cm
Lymphoma infiltration: [yes/no]
  If yes: **infiltration pattern:** [diffuse/miliary lesions/nodules/solitary mass]; **location:** [ ]
FDG uptake: [SUVmax]
Bone marrow:
Lymphoma infiltration: [yes/no]
  If yes: **infiltration pattern:** [unifocal/multifocal/diffuse]; **location:** [ ]
FDG uptake: [SUVmax]
Biopsy feasible: [yes/no]
  If yes: **recommended biopsy site:** [ ] (▶ Fig. 5.1)
Other organs:
Lymphoma infiltration: [yes/no]
If yes: **affected organs:**
  - **Stomach:** [yes/no]
  - **Liver:** [yes/no]
  - **Lung/Pleura:** [yes/no]
  - **Kidney:** [yes/no]
  - **Central nervous system:** [yes/no]
  - **Skin:** [yes/no]

If yes: **infiltration pattern:** [diffuse/miliary lesions/nodules/solitary mass]; **index lesion specification**
(▶ Table 5.1)
Clinically significant non-lymphoma-related findings[1]: [ ]

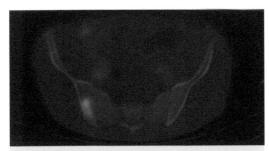

Fig. 5.1 Lymphoma infiltrating the right iliac bone. The report provides recommendation for the biopsy site.

5.2 Stakeholders

Clinical and radiation oncology specialists.

5.3 Pearls

- Positron emission tomography–computed tomography (PET-CT) imaging is considered standard for fluorodeoxyglucose (18F)-avid lymphomas like Hodgkin's lymphoma (HL), diffuse large B-cell lymphoma (DLBCL) (▶ Fig. 5.2), follicular lymphoma (FL), mantle cell lymphoma (MCL), and Burkitt lymphoma (BL),

Table 5.1 Index lesion specification

No.	Size (mm) (long-axis diameter) × (short-axis diameter)	FDG uptake (SUVmax)	Location (lymph node location/location within the affected organ)
1.			
2.			
...			

Table 5.2 Revised staging system[2]

Stage	Involvement	Extranodal status (E)
Limited		
Stage I	One node or group of adjacent nodes	Single extranodal lesion without nodal involvement
Stage II	Two or more nodal groups on the same side of the diaphragm	Stage I or II by nodal extent with limited, contiguous extranodal involvement
Stage II bulky[a]	II as above with bulky disease	N/A
Advanced		
Stage III	Nodes on both sides of the diaphragm Nodes above the diaphragm with spleen involvement	N/A
Stage IV	Additional noncontiguous extranodal involvement	N/A

[a]Whether stage II bulky disease is treated as limited or advanced disease may be determined by histology and a number of prognostic factors.

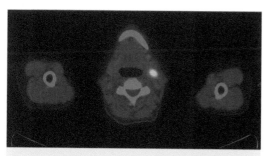

Fig. 5.2 Follicular lymphoma (indolent) transforming into diffuse large B-cell lymphoma (aggressive).

whereas CT is indicated for nonavid ones like mucosa-associated lymphoid tissue (MALT) or chronic lymphocytic leukemia/small lymphocytic lymphoma (CLL/SLL).[3]

- If PET-CT is performed in HL, bone marrow biopsy is no longer indicated.[3] It is only needed in DLBCL cases where PET-CT is negative and a discordant histology would directly impact patient management.

- For staging purposes a modified Ann Arbor staging system is recommended (▸ Table 5.2). Stages I and II are considered limited disease whereas III and IV are advanced one leading to different treatment options.
- Tonsils, Waldeyer's ring, and spleen are considered nodal tissue; (S) stands for spleen involvement, (E) for extranodal disease.
- Lesions should be measured in two dimensions: LDi (long-axis diameter) and SDi (short-axis diameter). They should represent overall disease burden.
- Nodal site is measurable if LDi > 1.5 cm, extranodal—if LDi > 1.0 cm.
- Splenomegaly is defined as spleen craniocaudal size > 13 cm.
- Bulky disease in HL has been defined as a nodal mass of 10 cm or greater than one-third of the thoracic diameter at any level of thoracic vertebrae. For FL, the cut-off value of 6 cm has been suggested and for DLBCL 6 to 10 cm. It is recommended to record the longest measurement by CT scan making the term (X) redundant.

- In a clinical trial setting it is recommended to report up to 6 index lesions (measurable nodal and extranodal) and up to 10 nonindex lesions representing the rest of the disease.
- Some indolent lymphomas, e.g., FL, can transform into aggressive ones like DLBCL characterized by a markedly higher FDG uptake, (▶ Fig. 5.2) directly affecting patient management.
- False-positive results may be caused by physiological uptake in: Waldeyer's ring, thymus, intestine, adnexa, or due to brown adipose tissue activation.
- Misdiagnosis may also occur due to high intestine activity (antidiabetic drugs), bone marrow activation (chemotherapy/granulocyte-colony stimulating factor [GCSF]), or lower uptake within the lesions (corticosteroid therapy).
- PET-CT quantitative methods (e.g., metabolic tumor volume [MTV] and total lesion glycolysis [TLG]) may improve visual assessment. They should be explored as prognostic factors and validated in further clinical trials.

References

[1] Niederkohr RD, Greenspan BS, Prior JO, et al. Reporting guidance for oncologic 18F-FDG PET/CT imaging. J Nucl Med. 2013; 54(5):756–761

[2] Cheson BD, Fisher RI, Barrington SF, et al. Alliance, Australasian Leukaemia and Lymphoma Group, Eastern Cooperative Oncology Group, European Mantle Cell Lymphoma Consortium, Italian Lymphoma Foundation, European Organisation for Research, Treatment of Cancer/Dutch Hemato-Oncology Group, Grupo Español de Médula Ósea, German High-Grade Lymphoma Study Group, German Hodgkin's Study Group, Japanese Lymphoma Study Group, Lymphoma Study Association, NCIC Clinical Trials Group, Nordic Lymphoma Study Group, Southwest Oncology Group, United Kingdom National Cancer Research Institute. Recommendations for initial evaluation, staging, and response assessment of Hodgkin and non-Hodgkin lymphoma: the Lugano classification. J Clin Oncol. 2014; 32(27):3059–3068

[3] Barrington SF, Mikhaeel NG, Kostakoglu L, et al. Role of imaging in the staging and response assessment of lymphoma: consensus of the International Conference on Malignant Lymphomas Imaging Working Group. J Clin Oncol. 2014; 32(27):3048–3058

6 Pancreatic Cancer Initial Staging Exam

Donald Kim, Susan Tsai, and Parag P. Tolat

6.1 Template

Pancreas:
Primary tumor:
- Size: [(AP × transverse × craniocaudally)] cm
- Appearance: [low-attenuation/hypervascular/cystic] mass
- Location: [head/body/tail]

Pancreatic duct: [dilated/not dilated], [ ] mm
[No other pancreatic mass is identified]

Mesenteric arteries:
Arterial anatomy: [normal (type I)/replaced right HA to SMA/completely replaced CHA to SMA]
Arterial tumor abutment or encasement:
- Celiac, common/proper hepatic, proximal splenic, left gastric and gastroduodenal arteries: [none/abutment (less than or equal to 180 degrees)/encasement (greater than 180 degrees)]
- Superior mesenteric artery (SMA): [none/abutment (less than or equal to 180 degrees)/encasement (greater than 180 degrees)]
- Other findings: [none or tumor abutment or encasement of additional arteries (i.e., inferior pancreaticoduodenal artery (IDPA), gastroduodenal artery (GDA), jejunal, middle colic, or ileocolic branches)]

Mesenteric veins:
Venous anatomy:
- Superior mesenteric vein (SMV) first jejunal branch: [posterior to SMA/anterior to SMA]
- Inferior mesenteric vein (IMV) drains into the [SMV inferior to the portosplenic confluence/central splenic vein]

Venous tumor abutment or encasement:
- SMV-PV-splenic vein confluence: [none/abutment (less than or equal to 180 degrees)/encasement (greater than 180 degrees)]
- First jejunal vein branch: [none/abutment (less than or equal to 180 degrees)/encasement (greater than 180 degrees)]
- SMV, PV, or segmental SMV-PV occlusion: [none]
- Other findings: [none or tumor abutment or encasement of jejunal, middle colic, gastroepiploic, or ileal branches of the SMV or long/short segment (approximately x cm) of tumor-free SMV inferior (caudal) to diseased segment]

Portal venous system: [normal and patent]
Inferior vena cava (IVC): [normal]

Hepatobiliary system:
Focal liver lesions: [none or describe lesions]
Biliary tree:
- Biliary stent: [none/plastic/metallic]
- Biliary dilation: [yes/no/describe]
- Common bile duct (CBD) diameter: [ ] mm

Gallbladder: [present/cholecystectomy]

Locoregional spread:
- Lymph nodes: [no adenopathy]
- Peritoneum: [negative, no nodularity or thickening/or describe lesions]
- Omentum: [negative, no nodularity or thickening/or describe lesions]
- Ascites: [none/mild/moderate/severe]

Other findings:
- Stomach, small bowel, and large bowel: [normal wall thickness, caliber, and enhancement/gastric outlet obstruction by tumor/duodenal outlet obstruction]
- Genitourinary system: [normal]
- Adrenal glands: [normal]
- Spleen: [normal]
- Lower chest: [normal]
- Bones: [no significant lesion]

Impression:
- Pancreatic [head/body/tail] mass measuring [ ] cm consistent with [pancreatic adenocarcinoma/neuroendocrine tumor/cystic neoplasm (describe type if possible)]
- [No metastatic disease]
- [No adenopathy]
- [No arterial or venous abutment or encasement]
- [Other impression statements]

6.2 Stakeholders

Surgical oncology, medical oncology, radiation oncology, gastroenterology, interventional gastroenterology, diagnostic radiology, interventional radiology, pathology, and research scientists.

6.3 Pearls

- Pancreatic cancer is the second most common gastrointestinal malignancy. Trends suggest that pancreatic ductal adenocarcinoma (PDAC) will become the second most common cause of cancer-related deaths by 2020.[1]
- Pancreatic cancer staging structured reports (SR) have been shown to provide essential information for consistent staging and treatment planning.[2]
- There are 12 key features which have been described as essential for adequate staging, with SR shown to report on 10.6 (+/– SD 0.9) of the 12 elements versus without SR, only 7.3 (+/– SD 2.1) of the 12 elements described.[2,3]
- Pancreatic cancer staging is based on tumor size, location in pancreas, tumor-vascular abutment or encasement, and metastatic disease. Only 15 to 20% of patients have potentially resectable disease at the time of presentation.[1]

- Various proposed clinical staging systems (▶ Table 6.1 and ▶ Table 6.2)[4,5] exist which categorize stage as: resectable, borderline resectable, locally advanced (type A vs. B), or unresectable/metastatic (▶ Fig. 6.1, ▶ Fig. 6.2, and ▶ Fig. 6.3). An agreed upon common staging system should be used for all key stakeholders at your institution and be reflected in the SR.
- Goals of surgery are to achieve R0 resection (negative margins), as positive margins are associated with poor long-term survival.[5] The SR will assist the surgeon in estimating the likelihood of R0 resection which may sometimes require portal venous or arterial vascular resection and reconstructions.
- Arterial and venous anatomical variants and tumor-vascular relationship descriptions aid surgeons in preoperative planning for vascular reconstructions, help prevent intraoperative anatomic misidentification, and avoid urgent, unplanned vascular resection and reconstruction.
- To adequately stage a tumor, a high-quality dual-phase pancreas protocol computed tomography (CT) and/or pancreatic magnetic resonance (MR) is required. Single-phase CT or bad quality exams may make it impossible to describe all the required elements to properly stage a tumor.[4]

Table 6.1 NCCN criteria for defining resectability status

Resectability	Arterial	Venous
Resectable	No arterial tumor contact (celiac artery, superior mesenteric artery, or common hepatic artery)	No tumor contact with the superior mesenteric vein or portal vein or ≤ 180 degrees contact without vein contour irregularity
Borderline resectable	*Pancreatic head/uncinate process* • Solid tumor contact with common hepatic artery without extension to celiac artery or hepatic artery bifurcation allowing for safe and complete resection and reconstruction • Solid tumor contact with the superior mesenteric artery of ≤ 180 degrees • Solid tumor contact with variant arterial anatomy and the presence and degree of tumor contact should be noted if present as it may affect surgical planning *Pancreatic body/tail* • Solid tumor contact with the celiac artery of ≤ 180 degrees • Solid tumor contact with the celiac artery of > 180 degrees without involvement of the aorta and with intact and uninvolved gastroduodenal artery, thereby permitting a modified Appleby procedure	• Solid tumor contact with the superior mesenteric vein or portal vein of > 180 degrees, contact of ≤ 180 degrees with contour irregularity of the vein or thrombosis of the vein but with suitable vessel proximal and distal to the site of involvement allowing for safe and complete resection and vein reconstruction • Solid tumor contact with the inferior vena cava
Unresectable	• Distant metastasis (including nonregional lymph node metastasis) *Head/uncinate process* • Solid tumor contact with superior mesenteric artery > 180 degrees • Solid tumor contact with the CA > 180 degrees • Solid tumor contact with the first jejunal superior mesenteric artery branch *Body and tail* • Solid tumor contact of > 180 degrees with the superior mesenteric artery or celiac artery • Solid tumor contact with the celiac artery and aortic involvement	*Head/uncinate process* • Unreconstructible superior mesenteric vein/portal vein due to tumor involvement or occlusion (can be due to tumor or bland thrombus) • Contact with most proximal draining jejunal branch into superior mesenteric vein *Body and tail* • Unreconstructible superior mesenteric vein/portal vein due to tumor involvement or occlusion (can be due to tumor or bland thrombus)

Source: Adapted from NCCN 2019.[5]

Table 6.2 Various definitions of borderline resectable PDAC

	NCCN definition	MCW definition	AHPBA/SSO/SSAT definition
Celiac artery		Abutment	No abutment or encasement
Common hepatic artery	Contact without extension to the celiac artery or hepatic artery bifurcation	Abutment or short segment encasement	Abutment or short segment encasement
Superior mesenteric artery	Contact ≤ 180 degrees	Abutment ≤ 180 degrees	Abutment ≤ 180 degrees
Superior mesenteric vein–portal vein confluence	Contact ≥ 180 degrees; Contact ≤ 180 degrees with contour irregularity or thrombosis with suitable vein proximal and distal to allow resection and reconstruction	Short segment occlusion that is amenable to resection and reconstruction	Abutment without impingement or narrowing, or encasement with/out short segment occlusion with suitable vein proximal and distal to allow resection and reconstruction

Abbreviation: AHPBA, Americas Hepato-Pancreato-Biliary Association; MCW, Medical College of Wisconsin; NCCN, National Comprehensive Cancer Network; PDAC, pancreatic ductal adenocarcinoma; SSAT, Society for Surgery of the Alimentary Tract; SSO, Society of Surgical Oncology.
Source: Adapted from Chatzizacharias et al.[4]

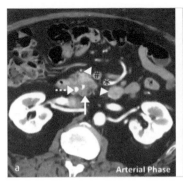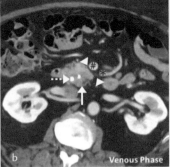

Fig. 6.1 (a, b) Resectable adenocarcinoma (subtle low-attenuation mass) of the pancreatic head/uncinate process (*arrow*). There is a normal fat plane (*arrowheads*) between the tumor and the superior mesenteric artery (SMA) (*) and superior mesenteric vein (SMV) (#). Note the mass is better seen on the pancreatic (arterial) phase. Plastic biliary and pancreatic duct stents are also present (*dotted arrows*).

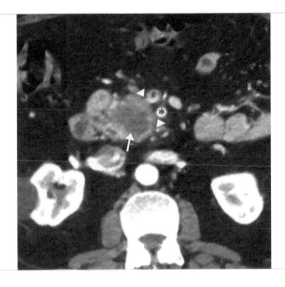

Fig. 6.2 Borderline resectable adenocarcinoma (low-attenuation mass) of the pancreatic head/uncinate process (*arrow*) with tumor abutment (*arrowheads*) of the superior mesenteric artery (SMA) (*) and superior mesenteric vein (SMV) (#). Note the low-attenuation soft tissue that abuts the SMA and SMV for less than 180 degrees and obliterates the expected normal fat plane.

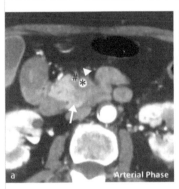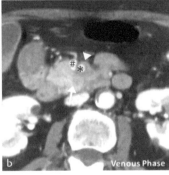

Fig. 6.3 (a, b) Locally advanced pancreatic adenocarcinoma of the uncinate process (*arrow*) with tumor encasement of the superior mesenteric artery (SMA) (*arrowhead*). Note the subtle low-attenuation mass in the pancreas (*arrow*) is better seen on the arterial phase. There is extrapancreatic soft-tissue (*arrowhead*) which encases the SMA (*) for 360 degrees and abutment with "tear-drop" shaped narrowing of the superior mesenteric vein (SMV) (#).

References

[1] Al-Hawary MM, Francis IR, Chari ST, et al. Pancreatic ductal adenocarcinoma radiology reporting template: consensus statement of the society of abdominal radiology and the American Pancreatic Association. Gastroenterology. 2014; 146(1):291–304.e1

[2] Brook OR, Brook A, Vollmer CM, Kent TS, Sanchez N, Pedrosa I. Structured reporting of multiphasic CT for pancreatic cancer: potential effect on staging and surgical planning. Radiology. 2015; 274(2):464–472

[3] Ter Veer E, van Rijssen LB, Besselink MG, et al. Consensus statement on mandatory measurements in pancreatic cancer trials (COMM-PACT) for systemic treatment of unresectable

disease. Lancet Oncol. 2018; 19(3):e151–e160–. Review. PubMed PMID: 29508762

[4] Chatzizacharias NA, Tsai S, Griffin M et al. Locally advanced pancreas cancer: staging and goals of therapy. Surgery. 2018; 163 (5): 1053–1062

[5] NCCN Clinical Practice Guidelines in Oncology—Pancreatic Adenocarcinoma. NCCN Guidelines, NCCN, 2019, www.nccn.org/professionals/physician_gls/pdf/pancreatic.pdf

7 Rectal Cancer

Doenja M.J. Lambregts and Regina G.H. Beets-Tan

7.1 Template

Primary Staging

Local tumor status:
- Morphology: [solid-polypoid/solid-(semi-)annular/mucinous]
- Circumferential tumor involvement: from [ ] to [ ] o'clock
- Distance from anorectal junction to lower pole of tumor: [ ] cm
- Relation to anterior peritoneal reflection: [below/above/crossing]
- Tumor length: [ ] cm
- T-stage: [T1–2/T3ab/T3 cd/T4]
  If T4, based on growth into: [ ]
- Sphincter invasion: [no/yes, internal sphincter only/yes, internal sphincter + intersphincteric plane/yes, internal + external sphincter]
  If yes, lowest part of invasion [upper/middle/distal] third of anal canal

Mesorectal fascia (MRF) involvement:
- Shortest distance between tumor and MRF: [ ] mm, indicating a [free (> 2 mm)/threatened-involved (≤ 2 mm)] margin
- Circumferential location of shortest distance between tumor and MRF: [ ] o'clock

Lymph nodes and tumor deposits:
- Total number of lymph nodes: [ ]
- Total number of *suspicious* lymph nodes: [ ], of which
  [ ] within mesorectum, [ ] extramesorectal
  Optional to include in report:
  ○ [ ] nodes with short axis ≥ 9 mm
  ○ [ ] nodes with short axis 5–8 mm and *at least 2* morphologic suspicious criteria
  ○ [ ] nodes with short axis 5 mm and *all 3* morphologic suspicious criteria
  ○ [ ] mucinous nodes (any size)
- N-stage: [N0/N +]
- Number of tumor deposits within the mesorectum: [ ]

Extramural vascular invasion (EMVI):
- Presence of EMVI: [yes/no]

7.2 Template

Restaging after Neoadjuvant Treatment

Local tumor status:
- Residual tumor mass: [no, completely normalized wall/no, fibrotic wall thickening without clear residual mass on T2W-MRI/yes, residual mass on T2W-MRI (and/or focal suspicious high signal on DWI)]

  If yes:
- yT-stage: [yT1–2/yT3ab/yT3 cd/yT4]
  If yT4, based on growth into: [ ]

- Distance from anorectal junction to lower pole of tumor: [ ] cm
- Relation to anterior peritoneal reflection: [below/above/crossing]
- Tumor length: [ ] cm
- Sphincter invasion: [no/yes, internal sphincter only/yes, internal sphincter + intersphincteric plane/yes, internal + external sphincter]

  If yes, lowest part of invasion [upper/middle/distal] third of anal canal

Mesorectal fascia (MRF) involvement:
- Shortest distance between tumor and MRF: [ ] mm, indicating a [free (> 2 mm)/threatened-involved (≤ 2 mm)] margin
- Circumferential location of shortest distance between tumor and MRF: [ ] o'clock

Lymph nodes and tumor deposits:
- Total number of residual suspicious (≥ 5 mm) lymph nodes: [ ], of which [ ] mesorectal and [ ] extramesorectal
- yN-stage: [yN0/yN +]
- Number of remaining tumor deposits within the mesorectum: [ ]

Extramural vascular invasion (EMVI):
Presence of EMVI: [yes/no]

7.3 Stakeholders

Members of multidisciplinary team involved in the treatment of colorectal cancer (radiologists, surgeons, gastroenterologists, medical and radiation oncologists, and pathologists).

7.4 Pearls

- Use of a structured report template is advised by the revised consensus guidelines on rectal magnetic resonance imaging (MRI) published by the European Society of Gastrointestinal and Abdominal Radiology (ESGAR) in European Radiology in 2018. The template described above is an adaptation of the ESGAR structured report template.[1]
- The items to be included in the structured report comprise the main discriminators used to determine the tumor risk profile and stratify patients into differentiated treatments (i.e., direct surgery for early stage tumors vs. preoperative short course radiotherapy or concomitant chemoradiotherapy for intermediate and locally advanced stage tumors).
- It has been shown that the implementation of structured report templates can significantly improve the quality of MRI reporting in rectal cancer and lead to higher satisfaction levels from referring clinicians.[2,3]

- The aim of T3-substaging is to categorize the depth of extramural tumor invasion with T3a indicating < 1 mm extramural invasion, T3b indicating 1- to 5-mm extramural invasion, T3c indicating 5- to 15-mm extramural invasion, and T3d indicating > 15-mm invasion. Increased extramural invasion depth is correlated with poorer prognosis. Tumors with an extramural invasion depth of < 5 mm (T3ab) on MRI have been reported to be associated with a good prognosis, similar to that of T2 tumors.[4]
- Imaging is well known to suffer from inaccuracies in nodal staging. Traditionally, mainly size criteria were employed, which led to overstaging of reactive nodes as well as understaging of small nodal metastases. The addition of morphological criteria (shape, border, signal heterogeneity) has been shown to improve accuracy.[5,6] The ESGAR guidelines acknowledge that—even with the addition of morphology—still no "perfect" criteria exist, but have adopted a set of practical guideline criteria (► Table 7.1 and ► Fig. 7.1) previously described in the national Dutch evidence-based guidelines on rectal cancer treatment. The main aim of adopting these criteria was to establish more stringent thresholds so as to avoid overstaging of nodes. In the Netherlands, adaptation of these criteria has led to a considerable increase in specificity for nodal staging with a consequent reduction in the

Table 7.1 Practical guidelines for nodal staging

Primary staging	
Criteria for N+	1. Short-axis diameter ≥ 9 mm (irrespective of morphology)
	2. Short-axis diameter 5–8 mm and ≥ 2 morphologically suspicious characteristics[a]
	3. Short-axis diameter < 5 mm and 3 morphologically suspicious characteristics[a]
	4. Mucinous node (any size)
Restaging after neoadjuvant treatment	
Criteria for N+	Short-axis diameter ≥ 5 mm (irrespective of morphology)

Note: At the time of publication of the ESGAR consensus guidelines there was no evidence supporting specific alternative criteria for extramesorectal lymph nodes. The criteria described above were therefore–as a practical guideline–advised to be applied to both mesorectal and extramesorectal lymph nodes.

[a]Morphologically suspicious characteristics:

1. Round shape

2. Irregular border

3. Heterogeneous signal

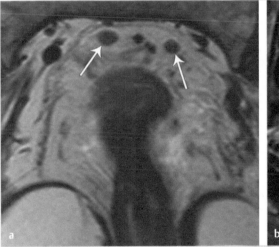 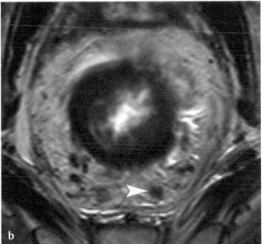

Fig. 7.1 (a, b) Examples of three similar sized lymph nodes (each falling in the size category 5–8 mm). Although the two nodes on the left image (*arrows*) have a round rather than oval shape, the two nodes do not fulfill the criteria for N+ nodes as they are regularly shaped and show a homogeneous signal. The small node on the right image (*arrowhead*) should be considered an N+ node as it has a round rather than oval shape, distinctly irregular border, and heterogeneous signal intensity.

(unnecessary) use of neoadjuvant radiotherapy for low-risk rectal tumors.[7]

- The anterior peritoneal reflection is an important landmark that is typically recognized well on MRI (▶ Fig. 7.2). Above the level of the anterior peritoneal reflection, the mesorectum is no longer enveloped by the mesorectal fascia anteriorly. Anteriorly, MRF invasion should therefore only be reported below the level of the peritoneal reflection. Above this level, the rectum is lined by the peritoneum anteriorly, which—if invaded macroscopically—would constitute T4a disease.

- Extramural vascular invasion (▶ Fig. 7.3) is increasingly acknowledged as an important prognostic staging factor although to date it is

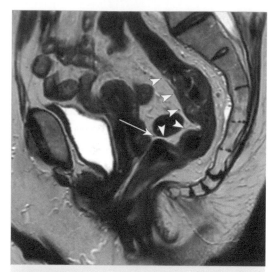

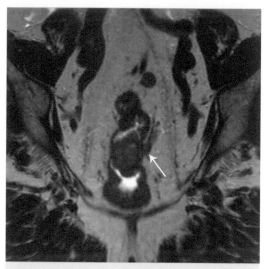

Fig. 7.2 Sagittal image of a female patient with a tumor in the upper rectum. The tumor is located above the level of the peritoneal reflection, which can be appreciated as a thin V-shaped line at the level of the cul-de-sac (*arrow*). Note, in male the peritoneal reflection is typically located just above the tip of the seminal vesicles. Above this level the mesorectum is lined by the peritoneum anteriorly (*arrowheads*). Although the tumor lies in close proximity to the peritoneum, there is no macroscopic invasion through the peritoneum; therefore, there is no risk for T4a involvement.

Fig. 7.3 Coronal images of a midrectal tumor showing clear extramural vascular invasion (EMVI) on the left lateral side (*arrow*). Tumors should be considered EMVI-positive if there is macroscopic extension of tumoral signal within an adjacent blood vessel with or without irregularity or expansion of the vessel contour.

not yet incorporated as a treatment determinant in the main clinical treatment guidelines.[8]

References

[1] Beets-Tan RGH, Lambregts DMJ, Maas M, et al. Magnetic resonance imaging for clinical management of rectal cancer: updated recommendations from the 2016 European Society of Gastrointestinal and Abdominal Radiology (ESGAR) consensus meeting. Eur Radiol. 2018; 28(4):1465–1475

[2] Sahni VA, Silveira PC, Sainani NI, Khorasani R. Impact of a structured report template on the quality of MRI reports for rectal cancer staging. AJR Am J Roentgenol. 2015; 205 (3):584–588

[3] Nörenberg D, Sommer WH, Thasler W, et al. Structured reporting of rectal magnetic resonance imaging in suspected primary rectal cancer: potential benefits for surgical planning and interdisciplinary communication. Invest Radiol. 2017; 52 (4):232–239

[4] Taylor FG, Quirke P, Heald RJ, et al. MERCURY Study Group. Preoperative high-resolution magnetic resonance imaging can identify good prognosis stage I, II, and III rectal cancer best managed by surgery alone: a prospective, multicenter, European study. Ann Surg. 2011; 253(4):711–719

[5] Brown G, Richards CJ, Bourne MW, et al. Morphologic predictors of lymph node status in rectal cancer with use of high-spatial-resolution MR imaging with histopathologic comparison. Radiology. 2003; 227(2):371–377

[6] Kim JH, Beets GL, Kim MJ, Kessels AGH, Beets-Tan RGH. High-resolution MR imaging for nodal staging in rectal cancer: are there any criteria in addition to the size? Eur J Radiol. 2004; 52(1):78–83

[7] Gietelink L, Wouters MWJM, Marijnen CAM, et al. Dutch Surgical Colorectal Cancer Audit Group. Changes in nationwide use of preoperative radiotherapy for rectal cancer after revision of the national colorectal cancer guideline. Eur J Surg Oncol. 2017; 43(7):1297–1303

[8] Chand M, Siddiqui MR, Swift I, Brown G. Systematic review of prognostic importance of extramural venous invasion in rectal cancer. World J Gastroenterol. 2016; 22(4):1721–1726

8 Prostate MRI

Benjamin D. Spilseth and Jeff Ames

8.1 Template

Indication:
Ideally includes prior biopsy type (TRUS, FUSION, IN BORE, date, and results), prior therapy (radiation, hormones)
Most recent prostate specific antigen (PSA):
Technique:
[State it is PI-RADS compliant; explicit description of field strength, coils used, type and dose of IV contrast administration. General description of pulse sequences performed, including b values for DWI]
Findings:
Size: L × W × H cm or V cubic cm (L*W*H*0.52)
Hemorrhage: [absent, mild, extensive]
Peripheral zone: [homogeneously hyperintense, heterogeneous, homogeneously hypointense] on T2-weighted images
Transition zone: [nonenlarged, enlarged with benign prostate hypertrophy (BPH) changes]
Lesion(s) in rank order of severity (highest score to lowest score, then by size): [ ]
1:
- Location: [right/left base/mid/apex peripheral zone/central zone] (IMAGE SERIES/NUMBER)
- Size:
- T2 description: [ ]
- T2 numerical assessment: [1–5]
- DWI description:
- DWI numerical assessment: [1–5]
- DCE description:
- DCE assessment: [positive/negative]
- Lesion overall PI-RADS category: [1–5]

Extraprostatic extension:
[No capsular abutment, capsular abutment < 6 mm, capsular abutment 6–15 mm, capsular abutment > 15 mm, capsular bulge or irregularity, gross extraprostatic extension]
Neurovascular bundles: description of proximity of any PI-RADS 4/5 lesion to NVBs
Seminal vesicles: [not involved by tumor]
Lymph nodes: [no adenopathy]
Bones: [no suspicious lesions]
Other pelvic organs: [no additional findings]
Impression:
- Based on the most suspicious abnormality, this exam is characterized as [PI-RADS 1/PI-RADS 2/PI-RADS 3/PI-RADS 4/PI-RADS 5]. The most suspicious abnormality is located at the [location] and there is [no evidence of extracapsular extension]
- No suspicious adenopathy or evidence of pelvic metastases

PI-RADS™ v2.1 assessment categories (▶ Fig. 8.1):
PI-RADS 1—Very low (clinically significant cancer is highly unlikely to be present)
PI-RADS 2—Low (clinically significant cancer is unlikely to be present)
PI-RADS 3—Intermediate (the presence of clinically significant cancer is equivocal) (▶ Fig. 8.2)
PI-RADS 4—High (clinically significant cancer is likely to be present) (▶ Fig. 8.3)
PI-RADS 5—Very high (clinically significant cancer is highly likely to be present) (▶ Fig. 8.4 and ▶ Fig. 8.5)

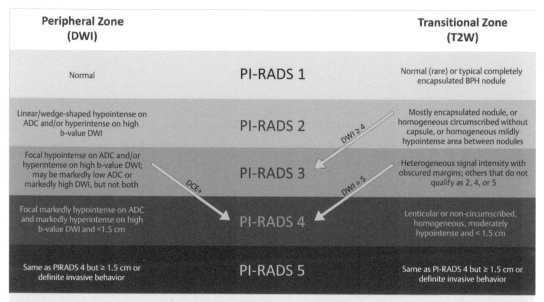

Peripheral Zone (DWI)		Transitional Zone (T2W)
Normal	**PI-RADS 1**	Normal (rare) or typical completely encapsulated BPH nodule
Linear/wedge-shaped hypointense on ADC and/or hyperintense on high b-value DWI	**PI-RADS 2**	Mostly encapsulated nodule, or homogeneous circumscribed without capsule, or homogeneous mildly hypointense area between nodules
Focal hypointense on ADC and/or hyperintense on high b-value DWI; may be markedly low ADC or markedly high DWI, but not both	**PI-RADS 3**	Heterogeneous signal intensity with obscured margins; others that do not qualify as 2, 4, or 5
Focal markedly hypointense on ADC and markedly hyperintense on high b-value DWI and <1.5 cm	**PI-RADS 4**	Lenticular or non-circumscribed, homogeneous, moderately hypointense and < 1.5 cm
Same as PIRADS 4 but ≥ 1.5 cm or definite invasive behavior	**PI-RADS 5**	Same as PI-RADS 4 but ≥ 1.5 cm or definite invasive behavior

Fig. 8.1 Simplified Prostate Imaging–Reporting and Data System (PI-RADS) v2.1 algorithm for determining the likelihood of malignancy in a given patient. The PI-RADS system classifies imaging features into very low (PI-RADS 1), low (PI-RADS 2), intermediate (PI-RADS 3), high (PI-RADS 4), and very high (PI-RADS 5) probability of prostate cancer. This classification relies on diffusion-weighted image (DWI) as the dominant sequence in the peripheral zone and T2-weighted image (T2WI) in the transitional zone. Note that positive enhancement in an otherwise PI-RADS 3 peripheral zone lesion increases that lesion to PI-RADS 4. Similarly, the DWI characteristics of PI-RADS 3 peripheral zone lesion can increase that lesion to PI-RADS 4. Similarly, the DWI characteristics of PI-RADS 2 and 3 lesions can increase the overall PI-RADS score.

8.2 Stakeholders

Urologic oncologists, urologic surgeons, abdominal radiologists, and radiation oncologists.

8.3 Pearls

- American College of Radiology Prostate Imaging–Reporting and Data System (ACR PI-RADS) is a reporting system for evaluation of prostate cancer, which is preferred by over 80% of radiologists and urologists.[1,2]
- In a recent survey, > 90% of radiologists and urologists preferred structured prostate magnetic resonance imaging (MRI) reports over free text.[2]
- Structured reporting has been shown to improve adherence with PI-RADS and may improve diagnostic performance for clinically significant cancer.[3] Published documented benefits of structured prostate MRI reporting include increased perceived clinical impact of report, improved reproducibility, and improved communication.[4,5]

- The above template is a modification of the ACR PI-RADS template which is also found on the ACR website. The PI-RADS template and this template were constructed based on surveys of radiologists and urologists.
- For instance, the majority of surveyed radiologists indicated that for prostate MRI, contrast dose and type, magnet strength, coil type, and any medications administered are essential report components.[2,6]
- The PI-RADS scoring system was updated in spring 2019 and is currently in version 2.1.[1]
- PI-RADS generates a score 1 through 5, ranging from very low to very high probability of cancer (▶ Fig. 8.1). The full PI-RADS reporting system description is available at https://www.acr.org/Clinical-Resources/Reporting-and-Data-Systems/PI-RADS.
- The transition zone is predominantly evaluated using the assessment of T2 W imaging. The peripheral zone is predominantly evaluated using diffusion-weighted image (DWI).
- The most recent update included minor changes in wording for characterizing lesions using DWI

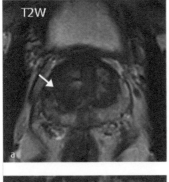

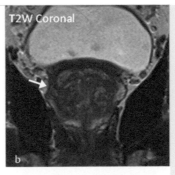

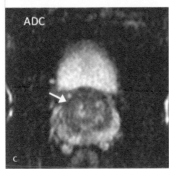

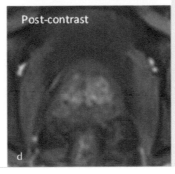

Fig. 8.2 (a–d) Prostate Imaging–Reporting and Data System (PI-RADS) 3. Small T2 hypointense lesion in the peripheral zone on the right base at approximately 9:00 position measures 6 × 6 × 4 mm (*arrow*). There is associated mildly decreased focal signal on apparent diffusion coefficient (ADC) map which was not hyperintense on high b-value diffusion-weighted images (not shown) and therefore does not meet PI-RADS 4 criteria. No corresponding abnormality is present on dynamic contrast-enhanced images, so this is classified as PI-RADS 3. This area was reportedly benign on biopsy, performed at an outside institution.

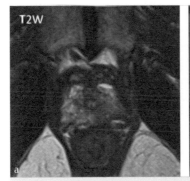

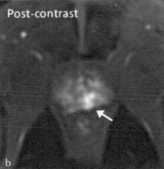

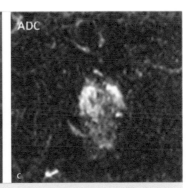

Fig. 8.3 (a–c) Prostate Imaging–Reporting and Data System (PI-RADS) 4. At 5:00 in the peripheral zone at the apex, there is a 1.2 × 0.8 cm focal area of decreased T2 intensity with associated substantial decreased signal on apparent diffusion coefficient (ADC) imaging indicating diffusion restriction (*arrow*). This lesion demonstrates rapid early focal enhancement with washout. No finding of extracapsular extension. Based on size < 1.5 cm and focal diffusion restriction, this is classified as PI-RADS 4. Biopsy demonstrated prostate adenocarcinoma with perineural invasion (Gleason grade 3 + 4). At prostatectomy, carcinoma involved approximately 10% of the prostate with perineural invasion and no extraprostatic extension.

affecting category 2 and 3 PI-RADS lesions. It also included changes to assessing category 1 to 3 lesions in the transition zone. There was no change from PI-RADS version 2 in category 4 and 5 lesion assessment.

- Following DWI assessment, peripheral zone PI-RADS 3 and 4 lesions may be distinguished utilizing dynamic contrast enhancement (DCE).

  ○ DCE is considered positive if focal early or contemporaneous enhancement is present correlating with a T2 or DWI abnormality.

- Transitional zone lesions assessed as PI-RADS 2 or 3 on T2 W imaging may be upgraded utilizing DWI.

  ○ DWI upgrades a transitional zone PI-RADS 2 lesion to a PI-RADS 3 lesion when there is a

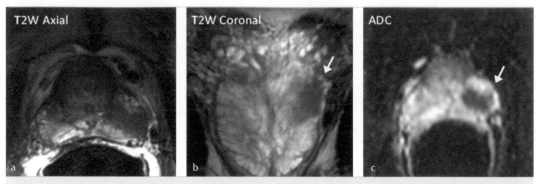

Fig. 8.4 (a–c) Prostate Imaging–Reporting and Data System (PI-RADS) 5 without extraprostatic extension. Large area of homogeneous decreased T2 signal in the left peripheral zone from the 2:00 to 4:00 position at the prostate base (*arrows*). This measures approximately 1.9 × 1.1 cm in greatest axial dimensions. It abuts the capsule for 0.9 cm without gross spread beyond the capsule, associated bulge, or irregularity, making it low risk for extraprostatic extension. There is associated marked restricted diffusion and abnormal early contrast enhancement. Due to diffusion restriction and size > 1.5 cm, it is characterized as PI-RADS 5. Initial histopathology revealed prostate adenocarcinoma (Gleason grade 3 + 3). Pathology after prostatectomy showed adenocarcinoma with areas of intraductal carcinoma involving 15% of the prostate (Gleason grade 4 + 4). Perineural invasion was present, without extraprostatic extension.

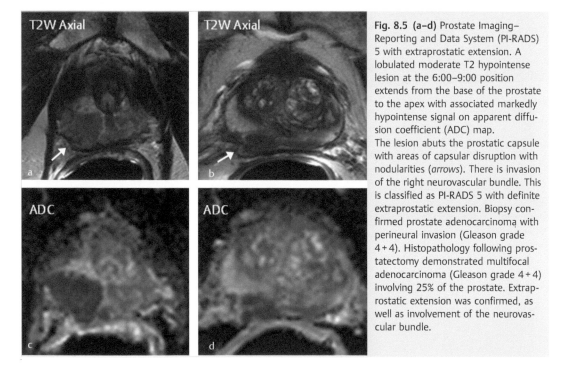

Fig. 8.5 (a–d) Prostate Imaging–Reporting and Data System (PI-RADS) 5 with extraprostatic extension. A lobulated moderate T2 hypointense lesion at the 6:00–9:00 position extends from the base of the prostate to the apex with associated markedly hypointense signal on apparent diffusion coefficient (ADC) map. The lesion abuts the prostatic capsule with areas of capsular disruption with nodularities (*arrows*). There is invasion of the right neurovascular bundle. This is classified as PI-RADS 5 with definite extraprostatic extension. Biopsy confirmed prostate adenocarcinoma with perineural invasion (Gleason grade 4 + 4). Histopathology following prostatectomy demonstrated multifocal adenocarcinoma (Gleason grade 4 + 4) involving 25% of the prostate. Extraprostatic extension was confirmed, as well as involvement of the neurovascular bundle.

DWI assessment of 4 or 5. This role of DWI is new in PI-RADS v2.1.

- DWI also upgrades a transitional zone PI-RADS 3 lesion to a PI-RADS 4 lesion when there is a DWI assessment of 5.[1]
- PI-RADS v2.1 also includes more information for identifying cancers in the anterior fibromuscular

stroma found at the anterior aspect of the prostate as well as in the central zone located as a pyramidal T2 hypointense structure in the base. For these regions, marked increased signal on heavily diffusion-weighted images as well as increased contrast enhancement is characteristic of malignancy.[1]

- An overall suspicion category should always be assigned for each lesion. Extenuating circumstances can be described as well (a lesion may be classified as a PI-RADS 4 but described as potentially compatible with prostatitis).
- Inclusion of management recommendations (biopsy recommendations, follow-up timing) is not preferred by most surveyed urologists.[2]
- Imaging specifications for MRI acquisition have been proscribed in PI-RADS, and the report should explicitly state that the exam was PI-RADS compliant.[1]
- Surveyed practicing radiologists prefer using image series and number, peripheral vs. central zone anatomy, and apex/mid gland/base terminology to localize lesions. Though recommended by PI-RADS committee, the PI-RADS sector map is generally not currently preferred in practice.[6]
- Use of specified lexicon to convey ideas such as levels of confidence in diagnosis of extracapsular extension may improve communication and help referring clinicians.[7] Most radiologists and urologists preferred verbal descriptions of confidence levels.[2]
- Length of capsular abutment has been shown to be more sensitive for the detection of extraprostatic extension than subjective assessments.[8,9]

References

[1] Turkbey B, Rosenkrantz AB, Haider MA, et al. Prostate Imaging Reporting and Data System Version 2.1: 2019 Update of Prostate Imaging Reporting and Data System Version 2. Eur Urol. 2019; 76(3):340–351

[2] Spilseth B, Margolis DJ, Patel NU, Ghai S, Rosenkrantz AB. A prostate MRI reporting: results from a survey of specialty societies. AJR Am J Roentgenol. 2017:(January): epub ahead

[3] Shaish H, Feltus W, Steinman J, Hecht E, Wenske S, Ahmed F. Impact of a structured reporting template on adherence to Prostate Imaging Reporting and Data System Version 2 and on the diagnostic performance of prostate MRI for clinically significant prostate cancer. J Am Coll Radiol. 2018; 15(5):749–754

[4] Magnetta MJ, Donovan AL, Jacobs BL, et al. Method to optimize prostate MRI. 2018:(January):1–5

[5] Faggioni L, Coppola F, Ferrari R, Neri E, Regge D. Usage of structured reporting in radiological practice: results from an Italian online survey. Eur Radiol. 2017; 27(5):1934–1943

[6] Spilseth B, Margolis DJ, Ghai S, Patel NU, Rosenkrantz AB. Radiologists' preferences regarding content of prostate MRI reports: a survey of the Society of Abdominal Radiology. Abdom Radiol (NY). 2018; 43(7):1807–1812

[7] Wibmer A, Vargas HA, Sosa R, Zheng J, Moskowitz C, Hricak H. Value of a standardized lexicon for reporting levels of diagnostic certainty in prostate MRI. AJR Am J Roentgenol. 2014; 203(6):W651–W657

[8] Mehralivand S, Shih JH, Harmon S, Smith C. A grading system for the assessment of risk of extraprostatic extension of prostate cancer at multiparametric MRI. 2018. doi: 10.1148/radiol.2018181278

[9] Rosenkrantz AB, Shanbhogue AK, Wang A, Kong MX, Babb JS, Taneja SS. Length of capsular contact for diagnosing extraprostatic extension on prostate MRI: assessment at an optimal threshold. J Magn Reson Imaging. 2016; 43(4):990–997

9 Renal Mass MRI and CT

Eric M. Hu, Nicole E. Curci, and Matthew S. Davenport

9.1 Template

Indeterminate Renal Mass Reporting:

The following core and optional renal mass reporting templates were designed by the Society of Abdominal Radiology Disease-Focused Panel on Renal Cell Carcinoma.[1,2,3]

They are designed for reporting Bosniak IIF-IV cystic masses[4] and solid masses without macroscopic fat characterized at renal mass protocol computed tomography (CT) or magnetic resonance imaging (MRI). Simple cysts, benign Bosniak II cysts, and classic angiomyolipomas with macroscopic fat do not require template reporting.

The core template contains important elements for routine reporting[3,5] (▶ Table 9.1). The optional template contains optional elements that can be selectively considered for inclusion by individual practices[1,2,3] (▶ Table 9.2). Items in brackets are input variables; lists separated by slashes are input variable options.

9.2 Stakeholders

General and subspecialty radiologists, urologists, and primary care providers.

9.3 Pearls

- The core and optional templates were iteratively designed[1,2,3] to improve the accuracy and consistency of renal mass CT and MRI reports.

Table 9.1 The core template

Core renal mass template	Dictation pick-list
Mass size	[X] cm
Growth rate	Previously [X] cm on [most recent relevant comparison date] and [X] cm on [oldest relevant comparison date]
Mass type	[Cystic/solid/indeterminate]
Bosniak classification	[Not applicable (not a cystic mass)/Bosniak I (simple cyst)/Bosniak II/Bosniak IIF/Bosniak III/Bosniak IV]
Macroscopic fat	[Yes/no]
Solid enhancement	[Yes/no/equivocal]
Axial location	[Anterior/posterior/neither anterior nor posterior]
Craniocaudal location	[Upper pole/interpolar/lower pole]
Mass margins	[Circumscribed/infiltrative]
Capsular location	[≥ 50% exophytic, < 50% exophytic, endophytic]
Distance to the sinus fat or collecting system	[X] cm
Tumor thrombus (distal extent)	[No tumor thrombus/ipsilateral renal vein (no IVC extension)/IVC below diaphragm/IVC above diaphragm/into right atrium]
Bland venous thrombus	[Yes/no] (optional free text description to follow)
Lymph nodes	[Normal/possible nodal metastases/definite nodal metastases] (optional free text description to follow)
Metastases in field of view	[None/possible distant metastases/definite distant metastases] (optional free text description to follow)

Source: Reproduced with permission from Davenport MS et al 2019.[3]

Table 9.2 The optional template

Optional characteristics	Dictation pick-list
Necrosis	[Not applicable (cystic mass)/yes/no]
T2w hypointensity	[Not applicable (not an MRI)/yes/no]
Microscopic fat	[Not applicable (not an MRI)/yes/no]
Enhancement type	[Entire mass/septal/mural/nodular/no enhancement]
Length of tumor thrombus	[X] cm
Caval wall invasion	[Definite/possible/no]
Ipsilateral renal artery anatomy	[Free text description]
Ipsilateral renal vein anatomy	[Free text description]
Description of individual Bosniak features	[Free text description]
Favored histology	[Clear cell RCC/papillary RCC/fat poor angiomyolipoma/RCC (unknown subtype)]
Follow-up imaging recommendation	[CT/MRI/ultrasound] in [X] months

Source: Reproduced with permission from Davenport MS et al 2019.[3]

The goal was the parsimonious inclusion of essential and preferred report elements.

- Nontemplate renal mass CT and MRI reports fail to include many features considered essential and preferred by radiologists and urologists.[1,2]
- Macroscopic fat in a renal mass almost always indicates classic angiomyolipoma and is a reliably benign feature in the absence of calcification or invasive behavior.[6]
- Microscopic fat in a renal mass only can be diagnosed using dual-echo gradient-echo imaging at MRI. It is a feature of clear cell renal cell carcinoma, fat poor angiomyolipoma, and rarely non-clear-cell RCC subtypes. Unlike macroscopic fat, masses with microscopic fat cannot reliably be considered benign.[6]
- The Bosniak classification is an effective way to convey the risk of malignancy in a cystic renal mass.[4,7] In conjunction with clinical factors, the Bosniak classification is used to inform management decisions including active surveillance, surgery, and, in some cases, ablation.
- The minimum standard for renal mass reporting is to determine if a mass is solid, cystic, or indeterminate; if solid, one should state whether it contains macroscopic fat; if cystic, one should state the Bosniak classification (exception: simple cysts); and if indeterminate, one should state what should be done to classify it.[1,3,7]
- Nephron-sparing approaches to renal mass management are gaining in popularity. They can

preserve kidney function without negatively affecting recurrence risk or survival. The RENAL nephrometry score is used to objectively determine the surgical complexity of a renal mass (▶ Table 9.3).[5] Although the reporting template does not include the nephrometry score, many of the constituent components that are used to derive the score (e.g., distance to sinus fat or collecting system) are included.

- Historically, Bosniak III and IV cystic masses were treated with surgical approaches. There is increasing evidence that active surveillance of Bosniak III cystic masses and percutaneous ablation of Bosniak III and IV cystic masses are viable and safe management options.[7,8]
- Imaging characteristics that can be used in conjunction with other findings to predict renal mass histologic subtype (e.g., microscopic fat) or aggressiveness (e.g., T2w hypointensity) are included in the optional template. In the future, their role in renal mass management may become more central as management schemes are designed to predict which patients will benefit most from biopsy, surveillance, or intervention.
- The American Joint Committee on Cancer (AJCC) TNM staging system for renal cell carcinoma uses CT or MRI features to predict patient outcome, including mass size, mass extent (fascial invasion, adrenal invasion, venous invasion), lymph node involvement, and distant

Table 9.3 Renal nephrometry score

Component	1 Point	2 Points	3 Points
R (radius, maximal diameter) (cm)	≤4 cm	>4 but <7 cm	≥7 cm
E (exophytic/endophytic)	≥50% exophytic	<50% exophytic	Completely endophytic
N (nearness to collecting system/renal sinus) (mm)	≥7 mm	>4 but <7 mm	≤4 mm
A (anterior/posterior location)	No points[a]; see below		
L (location relative to polar lines)	Entirely below lower polar line, or entirely above upper polar line	Mass crosses upper or lower polar line	≥50% of the mass is across the upper or lower polar line(s), or the mass is entirely between the polar lines, or the mass crosses the middle of the kidney

[a]No points given. The letter "a" (anterior), "p" (posterior), or "x" (neither anterior nor posterior) is listed after the score to describe the anteroposterior location.
Source: Adapted from Parsons RB et al 2012.[5]

Table 9.4 AJCC TNM staging system for renal cell carcinoma

TNM designation	Detail
T-stage	
T1a	Renal mass is ≤4 cm
T1b	Renal mass is >4 cm and ≤7 cm
T2a	Renal mass is >7 cm and ≤10 cm
T2b	Renal mass is >10 cm
T3a	Renal mass invades renal vein or renal mass invades sinus fat
T3b	Renal mass invades inferior vena cava below diaphragm
T3c	Renal mass invades inferior vena cava above diaphragm
T4a	Renal mass directly invades adrenal gland, another organ, or Gerota's fascia
N-stage	
N0	No regional lymph node metastasis
N1	Regional lymph node metastasis
M-stage	
M0	No distant metastasis
M1	Distant metastasis

Note: If more than one T-stage characteristic applies, use the highest applicable T-stage.

metastasis. Comprehensive reporting should include relevant staging details (▶ Table 9.4). Prediction of sinus fat invasion is difficult with imaging.

- Percutaneous biopsy can guide treatment recommendations for solid renal masses, but it is of limited utility for cystic masses.

References

[1] Davenport MS, Hu EM, Smith AD, et al. Society of Abdominal Radiology Disease Focused Panel on Renal Cell Carcinoma. Reporting standards for the imaging-based diagnosis of renal masses on CT and MRI: a national survey of academic abdominal radiologists and urologists. Abdom Radiol (NY). 2017; 42(4):1229–1240

[2] Hu EM, Zhang A, Silverman SG, et al. Multi-institutional analysis of CT and MRI reports evaluating indeterminate renal masses: comparison to a national survey investigating desired report elements. Abdom Radiol (NY). 2018; 43 (12):3493–3502

[3] Davenport MS, Hu EM, Silverman SG, et al. Standardized report template for indeterminate renal masses at CT and MRI: a collaborative product of the SAR disease-focused panel on renal cell carcinoma. Abdom Radiol (NY). 2019. doi: 10.1007/s00261-018-1851-2

[4] Bosniak MA. The current radiological approach to renal cysts. Radiology. 1986; 158(1):1–10

[5] Parsons RB, Canter D, Kutikov A, Uzzo RG. RENAL nephrometry scoring system: the radiologist's perspective. AJR Am J Roentgenol. 2012; 199(3):W355-W359

[6] Schieda N, Davenport MS, Pedrosa I, et al. Renal and adrenal masses containing fat at MRI: proposed nomenclature by the Society of Abdominal Radiology Disease-Focused Panel on renal cell carcinoma. J Magn Reson Imaging. 2019; 49 (4):917–926

[7] Silverman SG, Pedrosa I, Ellis JH, et al. Bosniak classification of cystic renal masses, version 2019: an update proposal and needs assessment. Radiology. 2019; 292(2):475–488

[8] Schoots IG, Zaccai K, Hunink MG, Verhagen PCMS. Bosniak classification for complex renal cysts reevaluated: a systematic review. J Urol. 2017; 198(1):12–21

10 Hepatocellular Carcinoma: LI-RADS and OPTN

Thomas W. Loehfelm and Victoria Chernyak

10.1 Template

Clinical information:
Etiology of cirrhosis: [toxic or metabolic, including EtOH/chronic hepatitis B/congenital hepatic fibrosis (LI-RADS v2018 does not apply)/vascular (LI-RADS v2018 does not apply)/other:]
Most recent AFP: [ ] ng/mL [date]
Highest AFP: [ ] ng/mL [date]
Treatment summary:
Targeted ablation:
[date]: [segment], [preablation size] [preablation LI-RADS category]
Local-regional:
[date]: [treatment] [targeted segments or lobes]
Systemic:
[start date] – [end date] [regimen]
Liver:
The liver is [cirrhotic/not cirrhotic]. The background liver parenchyma is [homogeneous/heterogeneous but not nodular/extensively nodular].[Hepatic arterial anatomy.][Portal vein assessment.]
Untreated observations:
Observation #: [1/2/3/4/5]
- **Location:** segment [I/II/III/IVa/IVb/V/VI/VII/VIII/other (*describe*)]
- **Size:** [ ] × [ ] [mm/cm] (image # [ ], series [ ])
- **Tumor in vein:** [no/yes (*describe the involved vessels*)]
- **LR-M features:** [none/*list all that apply*]
- **Nonrim APHE:** [yes/no]
- **Threshold growth:** [yes/no/not applicable]
- **Nonperipheral washout appearance:** [yes/no]
- **Enhancing capsule appearance:** [yes/no]

Ancillary features:
- Favoring benignity: [none/*list all that apply*]
- Favoring malignancy: [none/*list all that apply*]

LI-RADS v2018 category: [LR-NC/LR-1/LR-2/LR-3/LR-4/LR-5/LR-TIV/LR-M]
Treated observations:
Observation #: [1/2/3/4/5]
- **Location:** segment [I/II/III/IVa/IVb/V/VI/VII/VIII/other (*describe*)] (image # [ ], series [ ])
- **Treatment modality:** [ ]
- **Treatment date:** [ ]
- **Pretreatment category:** [ ]
- **Pretreatment size:** [ ] [mm/cm]
- **Enhancement in a nodular, masslike, or thick irregular pattern:** [yes/no/equivocal]
- **Size of enhancing component:** [ ] [[mm/cm]/N/A]

Enhancement characteristics:
- Arterial phase hyperenhancement: [yes/no/equivocal/N/A]
- Washout appearance: [yes/no/equivocal/N/A]
- Other: [enhancement similar to pretreatment/N/A]

Category: LR-TR [nonviable/equivocal/viable] [size] [mm/cm] (pretreatment [LR1/2/3/4/5/M/TIV/path-proven, [size] [mm/cm])

Remainder of the abdomen:
There is [no] extrahepatic malignancy

10.2 Stakeholders

Liver transplant surgeons and program coordinators, hepatobiliary surgeons, hepatologists, interventional radiologists, diagnostic radiologists, and oncologists.

10.3 Pearls

- Hepatocellular carcinoma (HCC) is unique in that high-quality standardized imaging is *diagnostic* of the disease, usually obviating the need for biopsy. The radiologist's description of the tumor directly affects patient eligibility for organ transplantation.
- Liver Imaging Reporting and Data System (LI-RADS) v2018 applies only in adult patients at high risk for HCC due to cirrhosis, chronic hepatitis B, or current or prior HCC.
- LI-RADS v2018 *does not apply* in patients less than 18 years old, patients of any age with cirrhosis due to congenital hepatic fibrosis, or patients of any age with vascular causes of cirrhosis such as hereditary hemorrhagic telangiectasia, Budd–Chiari syndrome, chronic portal vein occlusion, cardiac congestion, or diffuse nodular regenerative hyperplasia.
- Organ Procurement and Transplantation Network (OPTN) classification applies to *all* liver transplant candidates.
- OPTN and LI-RADS criteria for definite HCC (OPTN 5/LR-5) are identical *except for* 10 to 19 mm observations with nonrim arterial phase hyperenhancement (APHE) and nonperipheral "washout" but no enhancing capsule or threshold growth. Such a lesion is:
  - Categorized as LR-5 (definite HCC) in computed tomography/magnetic resonance imaging (CT/MRI) LI-RADS v2018.
  - Does not meet criteria for OPTN class 5.
- CT or MRI (▶ Fig. 10.1) scans used for model for end-stage liver disease (MELD) or pediatric end-stage liver disease (PELD) score exception requests must be interpreted by a radiologist at a transplant center.
- Report up to five individual observations with the highest LI-RADS categories. In patients with number of observations greater than five, the observations may be reported in aggregate to maintain report clarity.
- Assignment of the observation number should remain consistent across all examinations (i.e., observation designated as #1 should be labeled as #1 on all subsequent studies).

- Untreated lesion size is the single longest dimension, measured in any plane, including the enhancing "capsule" in the measurement, if present. Avoid size measurement on the arterial phase (AP) and diffusion-weighted imaging (DWI) if the observation is visible on other sequences/phases, due to perilesional enhancement on AP and potential distortion on DWI, which can affect the accuracy of the measurement.
- Viable tumor size after treatment should be measured as the longest dimension of the enhancing area of the treated lesion that does not traverse nonenhancing tissue, measured on the late arterial or portal venous phase.
- Threshold growth requires CT or MRI examinations performed no more than 6 months apart. If two exams are greater than 6 months apart, then growth of *any* magnitude is subthreshold. This includes new lesions on the current exam where previously there were none.
- Application of the ancillary features (AF) is optional but encouraged. If applied, the LI-RADS category can be upgraded by one if ≥ 1 AF of malignancy is/are present, and downgraded by one if ≥ 1 AF of benignity is/are present. The category should not be adjusted if AFs of both malignancy and benignity are present.
- If unsure between two LI-RADS diagnostic categories, choose the category reflecting lower certainty of the diagnosis:
  - If unsure between LR-1 and LR-2, choose LR-2 because that indicates a lower certainty of benignity.
  - If unsure between LR-4 and LR-3, choose LR-3 because that indicates a lower certainty of malignancy.
  - If unsure between LR-5 and LR-M, choose LR-M because that indicates a lower certainty of hepatocellular origin.
- Biopsy may be indicated for certain observations, either because of patient history, specific observation characteristics that lead to less confident diagnosis (i.e., LR-4 or LR-M lesions), or physician preference.
- If a specific lesion has a known pathology diagnosis, that diagnosis should be provided, and that specific lesion should no longer receive LI-RADS categorization. The exception to this rule is whether the pathology reports a hepatocellular lesion known to be a precursor of HCC (e.g., high-grade dysplastic nodule). In such cases, change in imaging characteristics and LI-RADS category should be reported as they can

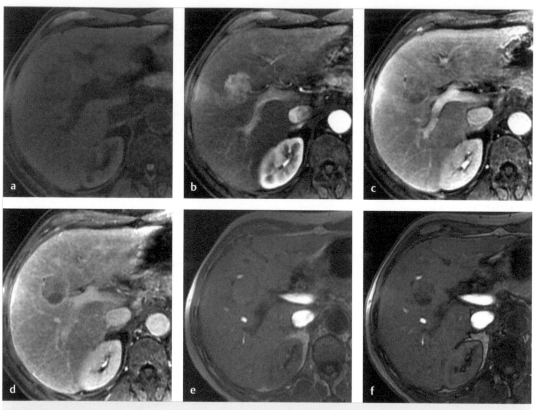

Fig. 10.1 Dynamic contrast-enhanced (**a–d**) and in- and opposed-phase magnetic resonance imaging (MRI) (**e, f**) shows a lesion at the junction of segments V and VIII. A comprehensive report would note that this patient has well-compensated cirrhosis due to alcohol abuse. Alpha fetoprotein (AFP) has not been measured yet and he has received no treatment for hepatocellular carcinoma (HCC). His liver parenchyma is heterogeneous but not nodular, and he has mild morphologic changes of cirrhosis but no evidence of portal hypertension. There is no extrahepatic malignancy. He has conventional hepatic artery anatomy. The lesion is reported as:

Untreated Observations:
Observation #: 1
Location: Junction of segments V and VIII
Size: 30 × 30 mm (image # 7, series 1303)
Tumor in vein: No
LR-M features: None
Nonrim arterial phase hyperenhancement (APHE): Yes
Threshold growth: Not applicable
Nonperipheral washout appearance: Yes
Enhancing capsule appearance: Yes
Ancillary features:
Favoring benignity: None
Favoring malignancy: Mosaic appearance, intralesional fat
LI-RADS v2018 Category: LR-5 (definite HCC)

signal progression to a frankly malignant lesion (► Table 10.1).

- LR-1 and LR-2 observations can be reported in aggregate—they need not be individually described. They should be reported in the impression *only if* they were a suspicious nodule on an antecedent ultrasound or if they are being

downgraded from a prior LR-4, LR-5, or LR-M categories, in which case explicit rationale for downgrade should be provided.

- LR-3 observations should be reported in the impression if there are no higher category observations, or if they are being downgraded from a prior higher category.

Table 10.1 LI-RADS category table

CT/MRI diagnostic category (treatment-naïve)	Explanation
LR-NC	Not categorizable due to image degradation or omission
LR-TIV	Definite tumor in vein
LR-M	Probably or definitely malignant, not HCC specific
LR-1	Definitely benign
LR-2	Probably benign
LR-3	Intermediate probability of malignancy
LR-4	Probable HCC
LR-5	Definite HCC
CT/MR treatment response category	**Explanation**
LR-TR nonevaluable	Treatment response cannot be evaluated due to image degradation or omission
LR-TR nonviable	Probably or definitely not viable
LR-TR equivocal	Equivocally viable
LR-TR viable	Probably or definitely viable

Abbreviation: HCC, hepatocellular carcinoma

- LR-NC (noncategorizable) or LR-TR nonevaluable categories must be reported in the Findings and Impression. The technical reasons for such categorization (e.g., omission of a required imaging phase) should be reported, and a recommendation for further work-up (e.g., repeat imaging with a different modality) should be provided.

Suggested Readings

American College of Radiology (2018). CT/MRI LI-RADS v2018 core. https://www.acr.org/-/media/ACR/Files/RADS/LI-RADS/LI-RADS-2018-Core.pdf

American College of Radiology. (2018). CT/MRI LI RADS v2018 manual. Chapter 14. LI-RADS reporting. https://www.acr.org/-/media/ACR/Files/Clinical-Resources/LIRADS/Chapter-14-LIR-ADS-reporting.pdf?la=en

Flusberg M, Ganeles J, Ekinci T, et al. Impact of structured report template on the quality of CT and MRI reports for hepatocellular carcinoma diagnosis. J Am Coll Radiol. 2017; 14(9):1206–1211

Organ Procurement and Transplantation Network. (2019). Policies. https://optn.transplant.hrsa.gov/governance/policies

Poullos PD, Tseng JJ, Melcher ML, et al. Structured reporting of multiphasic CT for hepatocellular carcinoma: effect on staging and suitability for transplant. AJR Am J Roentgenol. 2018; 210(4): 766–774

11 Hilar Cholangiocarcinoma

Anuradha S. Shenoy-Bhangle

11.1 Template

Morphologic evaluation:
- Tumor visible: [yes/no]
- Size (maximal axial dimensions in cm): [cm]
- Location (upper/mid/lower third of bile duct): [upper/mid/lower third]

Bile duct evaluation:
- Hepatic duct involvement: [right/left/both]
- Second-order ductal branch involved and side: [yes/no; right/left]

Arterial evaluation:
- Common/hepatic artery proper involvement: [present/absent]
- Solid soft tissue contact: [< /=/ > 180 degrees]
- Focal vessel narrowing or contour irregularity
- Aberrant/accessory arterial anatomy: (yes/no—specify)
- Solid soft tissue contact: (< / = 180 degrees)
- Focal vessel narrowing or contour irregularity

Venous evaluation:
- Portal vein involvement: [yes/no—main/right/left]
- Solid soft tissue contact: [< /=/ > 180 degrees]
- Focal vessel narrowing or contour irregularity
- Venous variants: [refer below]
- **Lymph nodal enlargement** [> 1 cm short axis]: [yes/no—number of enlarged nodes]
- [N1: LNds along: cystic duct, common bile duct, proper hepatic artery, portal vein]
- [N2: LNds: periaortic, pericaval, celiac artery, and SMA]

Surgically important bile duct and vascular variants:
Portal venous variants: PV trifurcation; right posterior branch from MPV; right anterior branch from MPV; complete absence of RPV; short LPV
Hepatic venous variants: SegVIII hepatic vein into middle hepatic vein; segments V and VI accessory inferior hepatic veins directly into the IVC; accessory middle hepatic directly into IVC
Hepatic artery variants: Replaced common/right/left hepatic artery; accessory right/left hepatic artery
Bile duct variants: Trifurcation; short right hepatic duct; right anterior hepatic duct draining into common hepatic; right posterior duct into left hepatic duct; right anterior duct into left hepatic duct
Remnant liver volume: [As per local surgeon preference]
Distant metastases: Mention as observed

11.2 Stakeholders

Hepatic and transplant surgeons, oncologists, and interventional radiologists.

11.3 Pearls

- Currently, surgical resection is the only curative treatment option for long-term survival and cure.

- There is no unified classification system for accurate presurgical staging of hilar cholangiocarcinoma. Various systems used include Bismuth–Corlette (BC); American Joint Commission on Cancer (AJCC)-Tumor, Node Metastases (TNM); Memorial Sloan Kettering Cancer Center (MSKCC), and the most recent by Deoliveira et al.
- The Bismuth–Corlette classification system (▶ Table 11.1) is the most popular with

surgeons. As a general guideline, type I and II undergo hilar resection, type III are treated with major hepatectomy, and type IV are considered unresectable. However, this system does not take into account vascular structures, lymph nodes, or metastases, which are described by the other systems described above.

- Multiphase computed tomography (CT) and magnetic resonance imaging (MRI) with magnetic resonance cholangiopancreatography (MRCP) both provide complementary information useful for accurate preoperative planning. Imaging for staging should be performed prior to biliary intervention (▶ Fig. 11.1).
- Besides Bismuth type IV, imaging findings that deem a hilar cholangiocarcinoma unresectable include bilateral hepatic arterial encasement; occlusion/encasement of the main portal vein; atrophy of one lobe with encasement of the contralateral hepatic artery; portal vein or second-order bile ducts; nodal metastases beyond the hepatoduodenal ligament or along the common hepatic artery (▶ Fig. 11.2).

- Future liver remnant (FLR) biliary drainage (if there is biliary obstruction) and portal vein embolization (if expected FLR is less than 30–40%) are helpful for remnant liver hypertrophy.
- Vascular involvement is indicated by loss of fat plane between the vessel and tumor (greater than 180-degree encasement, focal vessel narrowing, or contour irregularity).
- Mimics causing multifocal biliary obstruction include primary sclerosing cholangitis, Ig-G4-related sclerosing cholangitis, colorectal metastases.
- Nodes along the cystic duct, common bile duct, proper hepatic artery, and portal vein are considered regional lymph nodes while nodes in the periaortic, pericaval, superior mesenteric, celiac artery, or along the common hepatic artery are considered distant. Positron emission

Table 11.1 Bismuth–Corlette classification for perihilar cholangiocarcinomas

Type 1	Confined to the common hepatic duct below the confluence of right and left hepatic ducts
Type 2	Confluence of the right and left hepatic ducts
Type 3A	Type 2 + extension to bifurcation of the right hepatic duct
Type 3B	Type 2 + extension to the bifurcation of the left hepatic duct
Type 4	Extension to the bifurcations of both right and left hepatic ducts or multifocal involvement

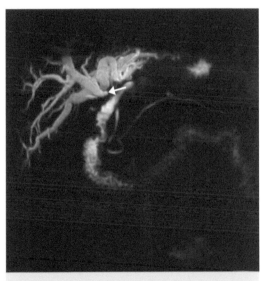

Fig. 11.1 Magnetic resonance cholangiopancreatography (MRCP) high-grade hilar stricture (*arrow*) caused by hilar cholangiocarcinoma with diffuse intrahepatic biliary ductal dilation.

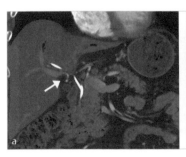 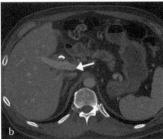

Fig. 11.2 Coronal arterial phase reformatted image demonstrates relationship of the hepatic artery proper to the hilar mass (*arrow*, **a**). The main portal vein is spared (*arrow*, **b**).

tomography-computed tomography (PET-CT) has more sensitivity to detect nodal disease than CT or MRI alone.

- Metastases to the liver, lung, peritoneum, bones, and adrenals should be sought for.

Suggested Readings

Engelbrecht MR, Katz SS, van Gulik TM, Laméris JS, van Delden OM. Imaging of perihilar cholangiocarcinoma. AJR Am J Roentgenol. 2015; 204(4):782–791

Deoliveira ML, Schulick RD, Nimura Y, et al. New staging system and a registry for perihilar cholangiocarcinoma. Hepatology. 2011; 53(4):1363–1371

Itri JN, de Lange EE. Extrahepatic cholangiocarcinoma: what the surgeon needs to know. Radiographics. 2018; 38(7):2019–2020

Joo I, Lee JM, Yoon JH. Imaging diagnosis of intrahepatic and perihilar cholangiocarcinoma: recent advances and challenges. Radiology. 2018; 288(1):7–13

Zhang H, Zhu J, Ke F, et al. Radiological imaging for assessing the respectability of hilar cholangiocarcinoma: a systematic review and meta-analysis. BioMed Res Int. 2015; 2015:497–942

12 Ovarian Cancer Staging

Jeanne M. Horowitz, Olga R. Brook, Elizabeth A. Sadowski, Edward J. Tanner, and Atul B. Shinagare

12.1 Template

Adnexal lesion: [right/left/bilateral] [cystic/solid/cystic with (mural nodule/papillary projection/irregular septation/large solid component)]
Invasion: [none/bladder/colorectal/pelvic sidewall/anterior abdominal wall/vessels] measuring [ ] × [ ] cm, series [ ], image [ ]
Ascites: [none/small/moderate/large]
Peritoneal metastases: [none/only in pelvis/in abdomen and pelvis] in the following sites: [largest greater omental deposit/cul de sac/paracolic gutter/subdiaphragmatic space/liver capsule/spleen capsule/porta hepatis/lesser sac-stomach/mesenteric root/serosal on small bowel/serosal on colon/ureters/umbilicus]
Lymphadenopathy: [none/only below renal arteries/above and below renal arteries] in the following sites: [internal iliac/external iliac/common iliac/retroperitoneal/mesenteric root/porta hepatis/splenic hilum]
Intra-abdominal stage IV disease: [none/liver intraparenchymal/spleen intraparenchymal/inguinal lymphadenopathy/bone/other]
Thoracic stage IV disease: [none/thoracic lymphadenopathy (size, location, and image)/pleural effusion (small/moderate/large)/pulmonary nodules (size, location, and image)]

12.2 Stakeholders

Gynecologic oncologists, medical oncologists, and pathologists.

12.3 Pearls

- This template applies for staging of ovarian, fallopian tube, and primary peritoneal cancer, which share similar molecular, imaging, and clinical features (▶ Table 12.1).[1]
- Most ovarian cancers present as stage III (84% are stage IIIC) and are high-grade serous carcinomas.[1,2] Twelve to 21% of patients with ovarian cancer present with stage IV disease.[2]
- Computed tomography (CT) with intravenous and oral contrast, in portal venous phase, is the most appropriate imaging exam for ovarian cancer prior to surgery and during treatment or surveillance (▶ Fig. 12.1a, b). Positron emission tomography-computed tomography (PET-CT) or magnetic resonance imaging (MRI) may be helpful for problem solving.[3,4]
- The anatomic sites and volume of disease can be used to determine if patients are good candidates for optimal cytoreductive surgery.[5] Cytoreductive surgery is considered complete if there is no visible residual tumor (R0), optimal if residual tumor is 1 cm or less (R1), and suboptimal if tumor nodules are greater than 1 cm.[1,4,5]
- Peritoneal implants in the root of the small bowel mesentery and porta hepatis are most associated with suboptimal cytoreduction, as disease close to the root of the mesentery or large enough to cause mesenteric retraction is difficult to resect safely.[5]
- Other sites of disease that may signal complex or suboptimal cytoreduction include suprarenal para-aortic lymph nodes >1 cm, implants in the lesser sac, gastrosplenic ligament, Morrison's pouch, gallbladder fossa, falciform ligament, or diaphragm.[1,4,5,6]
- Serosal implants can cause complications such as bowel obstruction, fistulas, or perforation, particularly during postoperative treatment.
- Lymph nodes in the abdomen and pelvis are considered involved if they have a short axis

Table 12.1 FIGO ovarian cancer staging 2014

	Location of tumor
Stage I	One or both ovaries
Stage II	Pelvic peritoneum, other than on ovaries
Stage III	Retroperitoneal lymph nodes or abdominal peritoneum
Stage IV	Malignant pleural effusion Distant metastases, including intrathoracic, intraparenchymal, and inguinal

Source: Adapted from Prat 2014.[8]

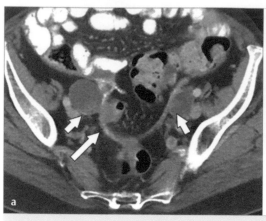
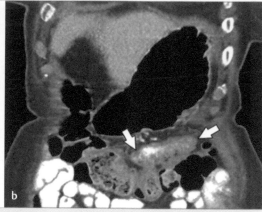

Fig. 12.1 (a, b) Eighty-two-year-old woman with high-grade serous papillary carcinoma. Axial (a) contrast-enhanced computed tomography (CT) shows peritoneal metastatic disease seen as pelvic peritoneal thickening with calcification (a, *long arrow*) and bilateral ovarian lesions suspicious for malignancy with solid and cystic components (a, *short arrows*). Omental caking in the transverse mesocolon on the coronal image (b, *arrows*) should be noted for the surgeon.

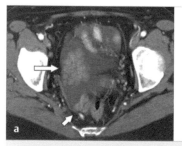
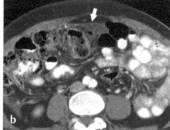
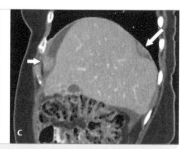

Fig. 12.2 (a–c) Sixty-three-year-old woman with papillary serous adenocarcinoma. Axial (a, b) and sagittal (c) contrast-enhanced computed tomography (CT) shows a predominantly solid right ovarian mass (a, *long arrow*), peritoneal tumor implants in the cul-de-sac (a, *short arrow*), omental caking (b, *arrow*), and peritoneal implants along the right diaphragm (c, *arrows*). Note that the tumor implant along the diaphragm causes impression on the liver capsule (stage III) and should not be mistaken for an intraparenchymal liver metastasis (stage IV).

greater than 1 cm or have abnormal morphology (round shape, heterogeneous enhancement or necrotic center).

- Hepatic and splenic parenchymal metastases (stage IV) need to be differentiated from invasion by peritoneal implants (stage III) as they have different prognosis[2,7] (▶ Fig. 12.2a–c).
- CT of the chest is commonly performed for ovarian cancer staging along with CT of the abdomen and pelvis to detect cardiophrenic and mediastinal lymphadenopathy, pleural effusions, and pulmonary metastases. Thoracic metastatic disease in ovarian cancer indicates stage IV disease.

- Ovarian cancer complications such as bowel obstruction, hydronephrosis, venous thrombosis, and pulmonary emboli are not specifically described in this template, but should be described in the imaging report, put in the impression, and communicated to the referring physician.
- Limitations of CT: Tumor deposits < 5 mm might not be seen, even when innumerable.[4,5] This can be a problem because small imaging-occult peritoneal implants completely coating the serosa of the small bowel or colon in the setting of large volume ascites will prevent optimal cytoreductive surgery.

References

[1] Javadi S, Ganeshan DM, Qayyum A, Iyer RB, Bhosale P. Ovarian cancer, the revised FIGO Staging System, and the role of imaging. AJR Am J Roentgenol. 2016; 206(6):1351–1360

[2] Heintz AP, Odicino F, Maisonneuve P, et al. Carcinoma of the ovary: FIGO 26th Annual Report on the results of treatment in gynecological cancer. Int J Gynaecol Obstet. 2006; 95 Suppl 1:S161–S192

[3] Schmidt S, Meuli RA, Achtari C, Prior JO. Peritoneal carcinomatosis in primary ovarian cancer staging: comparison between MDCT, MRI, and 18F-FDG PET/CT. Clin Nucl Med. 2015; 40(5):371–377

[4] Kang SK, Reinhold C, Atri M, et al. Expert Panel on Women's Imaging. ACR Appropriateness Criteria staging and follow-up of ovarian cancer. J Am Coll Radiol. 2018; 15(5S):S198–S207

[5] Sahdev A. CT in ovarian cancer staging: how to review and report with emphasis on abdominal and pelvic disease for surgical planning. Cancer Imaging. 2016; 16(1):19–19

[6] Qayyum A, Coakley FV, Westphalen AC, Hricak H, Okuno WT, Powell B. Role of CT and MR imaging in predicting optimal cytoreduction of newly diagnosed primary epithelial ovarian cancer. Gynecol Oncol. 2005; 96(2):301–306

[7] Tanner EJ, Long KC, Feffer JB, et al. Parenchymal splenic metastasis is an independent negative predictor of overall survival in advanced ovarian, fallopian tube, and primary peritoneal cancer. Gynecol Oncol. 2013; 128(1):28–33

[8] Prat J, FIGO Committee on Gynecologic Oncology. Staging classification for cancer of the ovary, fallopian tube, and peritoneum. Int J Gynaecol Obstet. 2014; 124(1):1–5

13 Endometrial Cancer MRI Staging

Stephanie Nougaret

13.1 Template

Uterus:
- The uterus is [anteverted/mid-positioned/retroverted] measuring [ ] × [ ] × [ ] cm
- Endometrial thickness is [ ] cm
- Tumor size is [ ] × [ ] × [ ] cm
- Cornual location: [absent/present]
- Myometrial invasion: [absent/superficial (< 50% of myometrial thickness)/deep (≥ 50% of myometrial thickness)]
- Uterine serosa invasion: [absent/present]
- Benign disease: adenomyosis: [absent/present]; leiomyomas: [absent/present]

Cervix:
- Cervical stroma invasion: [absent/present]
- Parametria invasion: [absent/present]

Vagina: [no invasion/tumor extend into the vagina/drop metastasis to vagina is present]
Ovaries: [normal/direct tumor extension into the ovary(ies)/metastasis to ovary(ies)]
Bladder/Rectum:
- Bladder invasion: [absent/present]
- Rectum invasion: [absent/present]

Lymph nodes:
[No pelvic adenopathy]/[pelvic adenopathy is present in [ ] locations measuring [ ] cm in short axis]
Other:
- Ascites: [none/small/moderate/large]
- Peritoneal implants: [absent/present measuring [ ] × [ ] × [ ] cm in [___] location [series [__], image [__]]
- See ▶ Table 13.1 for endometrial cancer staging

Table 13.1 2009 FIGO endometrial cancer staging

Stage	
I.	Tumor confined to the corpus uteri
IA.	No or less than half myometrial invasion
IB.	Invasion equal to or more than half of the myometrium
II.	Tumor invades cervical stroma but does not extend beyond the uterus
III.	Local and/or regional spread of the tumor
IIIA.	Tumor invades the serosa of the corpus uteri and/or adnexae
IIIB.	Vaginal and/or parametrial involvement
IIIC.	Metastases to pelvic and/or para-aortic lymph nodes
IIIC1.	Positive pelvic nodes
IIIC2.	Positive para-aortic lymph nodes with or without positive pelvic lymph nodes
IV.	Tumor invades bladder and/or bowel mucosa, and/or distant metastases
IVA.	Tumor invasion of bladder and/or bowel mucosa
IVB.	Distant metastases, including intra-abdominal metastases and/or inguinal lymph nodes

Source: Adapted from Creasman W, et al. Revised FIGO staging for carcinoma of the endometrium. Int J Gynaecol Obstet 2009;105(2):109.

13.2 Stakeholders

Gynecologic oncologists, radiation oncologists, and radiologists.

13.3 Pearls

- For assessment of deep myometrial invasion:
  - A high-resolution T2-weighted sequence in oblique plane perpendicular to the endometrial cavity is mandatory (▶ Fig. 13.1 and ▶ Fig. 13.2).[1,2,3]
  - An intact junctional zone and a smooth band of early subendometrial enhancement exclude deep myometrial invasion.
  - Deep myometrial invasion is suspected by the presence of low-signal-intensity tumor within the outer myometrium or beyond.[1,4]
  - Overestimation of depth of myometrial invasion may be caused by *adenomyosis*, *leiomyomas*, and *cornual tumor location*.[1]
- For assessment of cervical stromal invasion:
  - Cervical stromal invasion is diagnosed by intermediate- to high-signal-intensity tumor

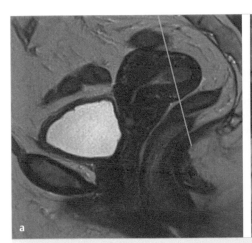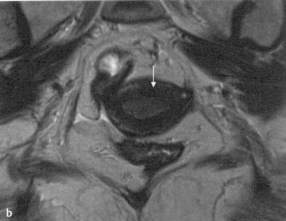

Fig. 13.1 Sagittal T2W image **(a)** in a postmenopausal patient shows a thickening of the endometrial cavity with an intermediate T2 signal mass. The white line on **(a)** represents the perpendicular axis of the tumor and axial plane required **(b)** to accurately evaluate deep myometrial invasion. Axial oblique T2W image **(b)** shows an intermediate T2 signal mass without deep myometrial invasion consistent with a FIGO IA tumor (*arrow*).

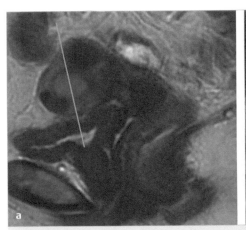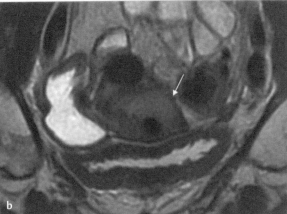

Fig. 13.2 Sagittal T2W image **(a)** in a postmenopausal patient shows a thickening of the endometrial cavity with an intermediate T2 signal mass. The white line on **(a)** represents the perpendicular axis of the tumor and axial plane required **(b)** to accurately evaluate deep myometrial invasion. Axial oblique T2W image **(b)** shows an intermediate T2 signal mass with deep myometrial invasion consistent with a FIGO IB tumor (*arrow*).

disrupting the normal low-signal-intensity cervical stroma.[3,5]

- ○ The presence of tumor extension into the endocervical canal or tumor widening the endocervical canal does not represent cervical stromal invasion.[5]
- For advanced cases:
  - ○ Disruption of the low-signal intensity of the uterine serosa and/or irregular uterine contour on T2WI, loss of the normal rim of highly enhancing myometrium on DCE indicate serosal involvement.[1]
  - ○ Magnetic resonance imaging (MRI) has low sensitivity for the detection of lymph node metastases. Diffusion-weighted imaging (DWI) aids in the detection of lymph nodes owing to their high signal intensity (SI) on high b-value images. However, it has a poor specificity to distinguish malignant and benign nodes.
  - ○ Bullous edema of the bladder may be a sign of tumor in the subserosal or muscular layer of the bladder, but this is not sufficient for diagnosis of bladder invasion. On T2WI, bladder/rectal involvement is diagnosed when tumor abuts or indents the bladder/rectum

over a significant area, interrupts the low-signal intensity of the bladder/rectal muscular layer, or invades the bladder/rectal muscular wall and tumor nodules are seen in the mucosal layer.

References

[1] Nougaret S, Horta M, Sala E, et al. Endometrial cancer MRI staging: updated guidelines of the European Society of Urogenital Radiology. Eur Radiol. 2019; 29(2):792–805

[2] Nougaret S, Lakhman Y, Vargas HA, et al. From staging to prognostication: achievements and challenges of MR imaging in the assessment of endometrial cancer. Magn Reson Imaging Clin N Am. 2017; 25(3):611–633

[3] Freeman SJ, Aly AM, Kataoka MY, Addley HC, Reinhold C, Sala E. The revised FIGO staging system for uterine malignancies: implications for MR imaging. Radiographics. 2012; 32 (6):1805–1827

[4] Beddy P, Moyle P, Kataoka M, et al. Evaluation of depth of myometrial invasion and overall staging in endometrial cancer: comparison of diffusion-weighted and dynamic contrast-enhanced MR imaging. Radiology. 2012; 262(2):530–537

[5] Cunha TM, Félix A, Cabral I. Preoperative assessment of deep myometrial and cervical invasion in endometrial carcinoma: comparison of magnetic resonance imaging and gross visual inspection. Int J Gynecol Cancer. 2001; 11(2):130–136

14 Cervical Cancer MRI Staging

Jessica B. Robbins

14.1 Template

Cervical tumor:
- Tumor morphology and site: [endocervical/exophytic/infiltrative], centered in the [anterior lip/posterior lip/circumferential]
- Tumor size: [ ] × [ ] × [ ] cm
- Distance from internal cervical os: [ ] mm
- Length of cervix: [ ] cm
- Uterine invasion: [absent/extending into[lower uterine segment/body/fundus]]
- Parametrial invasion: [none/unlikely/possible/present] in [position on a clock face] location
- Vaginal invasion: [none/upper two-thirds/lower third]
- Adjacent pelvic organs: [not involved/invades bladder/invades rectum]

Uterus:
- The uterus is [anteverted/midpositioned/retroverted] measuring [ ] × [ ] × [ ] cm
- Endometrium: [could not be identified/homogeneous/heterogeneous] measuring [ ] mm in dual thickness
- Myometrium: [normal/abnormal] [describe, if appropriate, including infiltrative tumor if applicable]

Ovaries:
- The ovaries are [normal/abnormal].
- Right ovary: [ ] × [ ] × [ ] cm [describe if abnormal]
- Left ovary: [ ] × [ ] × [ ] cm [describe if abnormal]

Lymph nodes:
- Pelvis: [none/few/many]; [if appropriate describe representative pelvic lymph node(s) location and short-axis size]. These lymph nodes are [unlikely/possibly/probably] malignant
- Para-aortic: [none/few/many]; [if appropriate describe representative pelvic lymph node(s) location and short-axis size]. These lymph nodes are [unlikely/possibly/probably] malignant

Other:
- Pelvic fluid: [none/present]
- Pelvic/Peritoneal implants: [none/present] [describe if appropriate]
- Hydronephrosis: [none/present] [describe if appropriate including right/left/bilateral, degree of dilatation, chronicity if possible to determine]
- Other findings: [none/present] [describe if appropriate]

14.2 Stakeholders

Gynecological oncologic surgeons and radiation oncologists.

14.3 Pearls

- Cervical cancer is staged according to the International Federation of Gynecology and Obstetrics (FIGO) cancer of the cervix uteri criteria. Historically, FIGO staging of cervical cancer was based mainly upon the clinical exam; however, the 2018 update of the FIGO criteria incorporates imaging and pathologic findings, when available[1] (▶ Table 14.1).
- Normal anatomy of the cervix is best depicted on T2-weighted images (▶ Fig. 14.1).
- While many tumors can be defined by the combination of T2-weighted and diffusion-weighted imaging (DWI), T1-weighted postcontrast images can confirm the extent of large infiltrative tumors. In addition, T1-weighted postcontrast images are helpful to determine if there is invasion of adjacent structures such as the urinary bladder or rectum (▶ Fig. 14.2).

Table 14.1 2018 Revised FIGO staging of cervical cancer

FIGO Stage		Description	Comments
I		Tumor is confined to the cervix	Extension into the myometrium does not alter stage
	IA	Invasive carcinoma diagnosed only by microscopy	Imaging occult
			IA1: stromal invasion < 3 mm
			IA2: stromal invasion 3–5 mm
	IB	Invasive carcinoma, stromal invasion ≥ 5 mm Tumor Limited to the cervix	IB1: tumor < 2 cm greatest dimension
			IB2: tumor 2–4 cm greatest dimension
			IB3: tumor ≥ 4 cm greatest dimension
II		Tumor extends beyond the uterus, but not into the lower 1/3 of the vagina or pelvic sidewall	
	IIA	Extrauterine extension limited to upper 2/3 of the vagina No parametrial extension	IIA1: tumor > 4 cm greatest dimension
			IIA2: tumor ≥ 4 cm greatest dimension
	IIB	Parametrial extension, but no pelvic sidewall involvement	
III		Tumor extends into the lower 1/3 of the vagina and/or pelvic sidewall and/or causes hydronephrosis and/or pelvic lymph nodes and/or para-aortic lymph nodes	
	IIIA	Extension to lower 1/3 of vagina without pelvic sidewall extension	
	IIIB	Extension to the pelvic sidewall and/or hydronephrosis or nonfunctioning kidney (unless known to be caused by something else)	
	IIIC	Involvement of pelvic and/or para-aortic lymph nodes, regardless of tumor size/extent	"r" (imaging) or "p" (pathology) notation indicated how lymph node involvement was determined
			IIIC1: Pelvic lymph node metastasis only
			IIIC2: Para-aortic lymph node metastasis
IV		Tumor extends beyond the pelvis or has invaded the mucosa of the bladder of rectum	
	IVA	Spread to adjacent pelvic organs	
	IVB	Spread to distant organs	

Source: Adapted from Bhatla et al (2018).[1]

- Since the *size of the cervical tumor* impacts the treatment strategy, accurate measurements are important. Bulky tumors, > 4 cm, are generally treated with primary chemoradiation.[2] Young women with small tumors, seeking to preserve fertility, may be candidates for radical trachelectomy if the tumor is < 2 cm, the overall length of the cervix is > 2.5 cm, and the tumor is > 1 cm from the internal cervical os.[2]

- Axial T2-weighted images, without fat saturation, are ideal for assessing the parametria. The intrinsically bright T2 signal of the parametrial fat provides inherent contrast to the dark T2 signal of normal cervical stroma and intermediate T2 signal of the cervical tumor. If the cervical stroma is circumferentially intact and the tumor is definitively confined to the cervix, parametrial invasion should be described as "none." If the tumor thins the cervical stroma and/or focally or diffusely expands the contour of the cervix but the parametrial fat is preserved, parametrial invasion can be described as "possible"; this alerts the surgeon to focus the physical exam in this region to determine if there is physical evidence of parametrial invasion. In the setting of lobular or infiltrative tumor extension into the parametrial fat and/or

encasement of parametrial vessels, parametrial invasion can be described as "present."[2,3]

- Obliteration of the T2 hypointense cervical stroma is indicative of parametrial extension (▶ Fig. 14.3). Parametrial extension can be overestimated with large tumors as secondary stromal edema can be misinterpreted as tumoral extension through the cervical stroma.[2]
- DWI should be used to confirm restricted diffusion within the tumor. DWI can increase conspicuity of small tumors and in the less common T2 isointense tumors as might be seen in younger women.[3]
- T1-weighted postcontrast images combined with DWI can be helpful in detecting extrauterine disease such as ovarian metastases or peritoneal implants.[2]
- Pelvic and para-aortic lymph node status is best assessed with a combination of T2-weighted and T1-weighted postcontrast images. Pathologic lymph nodes have a round morphology, are generally greater than 1 cm in short-axis diameter, and may be centrally necrotic. Lymph nodes with none of these suspicious features can be described as "unlikely" to be malignant, subcentimeter lymph nodes with a rounded morphology can be described as "possibly" malignant, and lymph nodes with a rounded morphology and short-axis diameter greater than 1 cm may be described as "probably" malignant.[2,3]

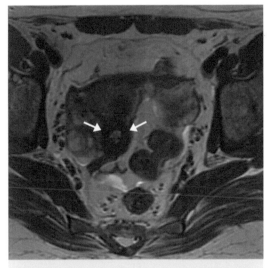

Fig. 14.1 Normal cervical anatomy. Axial T2-weighted without fat saturation. Normal cervical stroma is circumferentially dark in T2-signal (*arrows*).

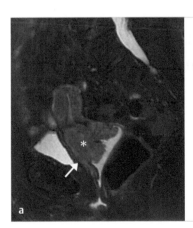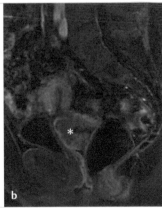

Fig. 14.2 Infiltrative cervical tumor. On the sagittal T2-weighed image (a), it is unclear if the tumor (*asterisk*) invades the bladder trigone (*arrow*); following contrast (b), the preserved plane between the bladder and the cervical tumor (*asterisk*) is more conspicuous.

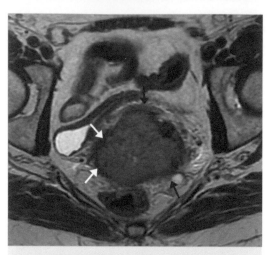

Fig. 14.3 Parametrial extension. The dark T2-signal cervical stroma (*white arrows*) is disrupted by the intermediate T2-signal tumor (*black arrows*) indicative of parametrial extension.

References

[1] Bhatla N, Aoki D, Sharma DN, Sankaranarayanan R. Cancer of the cervix uteri. Int J Gynaecol Obstet. 2018; 143 Suppl 2:22–36

[2] Sala E, Rockall AG, Freeman SJ, Mitchell DG, Reinhold C. The added role of MR imaging in treatment stratification of patients with gynecologic malignancies: what the radiologist needs to know. Radiology. 2013; 266(3):717–740

[3] Patel-Lippmann K, Robbins JB, Barroilhet L, Anderson B, Sadowski EA, Boyum J. MR imaging of cervical cancer. Magn Reson Imaging Clin N Am. 2017; 25(3):635–649

15 CT Staging Lung Cancer TNM 8

Julien Dinkel and Cornelia Schaefer-Prokop

15.1 Template

Procedure:
- CT technique: [low dose, IV contrast, PET-CT, etc]
- Image quality: [adequate, limited, etc.,]

Clinical information:
- Previous treatments: [surgery, chemotherapy, radiotherapy, immunotherapy]
- Histological type: [ ]
- Mutation: [ ]

Comparison:
- Modality: [CT, PET-CT, etc]
- Date: [ ]

Findings:
- Lung lesion(s):
  - Location: [parenchymal, perifissural, subpleural, endobronchial]
  - Appearance: [solid, part-solid, ground glass]
  - Affected lobe(s)
  - Size: [maximum diameter in one of the three planes in mm in lung window] (▶ Fig. 15.1). In a part-solid tumor, the size of the solid component determines the T stage
  - Infiltration of other structures: [aorta, pericardium, heart, bronchus, carina, diaphragm, pleura, mediastinal fat, mediastinal structures, etc]
  - Atelectasis or obstructive pneumonia
  - Satellite nodules: [same/other lobe, same/other lung]
- Lymph nodes
  - Affected regional lymph nodes: [based on IASLC stations]
  - Nonregional thoracic lymph node metastasis: [paracardial, internal mammary, intercostal, axillary, peridiaphragmatic, etc]
- Metastases
  - Intrathoracic metastases: [malignant pleural/pericardial effusion, contralateral lesion, lymphangitic carcinomatosis]
  - Extrathoracic metastases:
    – Number: [singular, multiple]
    – Location: [liver, bone, adrenal gland, lymph node, etc]
- Other findings [nononcologic]:
  - Structural lung changes [emphysema, fibrosis, etc]
  - Heart/large vessels
  - Nonmalignant findings in osseous structures
  - Abdominal organs as far as visible

Conclusion:
- T stage and invasion of surrounding structures:
  - T0 [no primary tumor on imaging]
  - Tis [< 3 cm pure ground glass]
  - Tmi [< 3 cm part-solid lesion with < 5 mm solid lesion]
  - T1 [≤ 3 cm]
    – T1a [≤ 1 cm]

- T1b [>1 to ≤2 cm]
- T1c [>2 to ≤3 cm]
  - T2 [3 cm to ≤5 cm or invasion of the visceral pleura, main bronchus, atelectasis, or obstructive pneumonitis extending to hilum]
    - T2a [>3 cm to ≤4 cm]
    - T2b [>4 cm to ≤5 cm]
  - T3 [>5 to ≤7 cm or invasion of chest wall, pericardium, phrenic nerve, or separate tumor nodule(s) in same lobe]
  - T4 [>7 cm or invasion of mediastinum (mediastinal fat), diaphragm, great vessels, spine, trachea, carina, esophagus, recurrent laryngeal nerve, or tumor nodule(s) in a different ipsilateral lobe]
- N stage
  - N0 [no suspicious lymph nodes]
  - N1 [ipsilateral peribronchial/hilar nodes]
  - N2 [ipsilateral mediastinal/subcarinal nodes]
  - N3 [contralateral mediastinal or hilar nodes; supraclavicular nodes]
- M stage
  - M0 [no evidence of metastasis]
  - M1a [intrathoracic metastasis (malignant pleural or pericardial effusion or pleural/pericardial nodules or separate tumor nodule(s) in a contralateral lobe)]
  - M1b [single extrathoracic metastasis]
  - M1c [multiple extrathoracic metastases]
- Further relevant findings

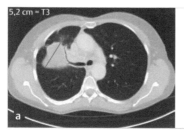 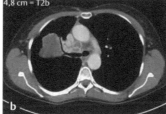

Fig. 15.1 **(a, b)** Correct measurement of lung lesions should be performed in lung window. The maximum diameter in either axial, coronal, or sagittal direction should be applied. This example shows a lesion with a diameter of 5.2 cm in lung window, which, therefore, represents a T3 tumor.

15.2 Stakeholders

Members of multidisciplinary team involved in the treatment of lung cancer (radiologists, nuclear medicine physicians, oncologists, pulmonologists, radiation therapists, and thoracic surgeons).

15.3 Pearls[1,2,3,4]

- To ensure an ideal clinical benefit for referring physicians, CT scans for staging of lung cancer should reflect the TNM classification in their structures and include respective subheadings (lesions/lymph nodes/metastases).
- The structured report should include all relevant information on the primary tumor necessary for a full T-staging, i.e., diameter and infiltration of surrounding structures. Infiltration is of

particular importance with regard to respectability (▶ Fig. 15.2).
- Measurement of lung tumors should be performed in lung window and on multiplanar reconstructions for accurate T-staging. In a part-solid tumor, the size of the solid component determines the T-stage.
- One or more satellite lesions in *the same* lobe are regarded as T3, whereas one or more ipsilateral satellite lesions in *another* lobe are classified as T4. Contralateral lesions are regarded as metastatic disease and therefore M1a.
- Suspicious lymph nodes' location should be reported according to the International Association of the Study of Lung Cancer (IASLC).
- In contrast to earlier TNM classification systems, for metastatic disease, a distinction between

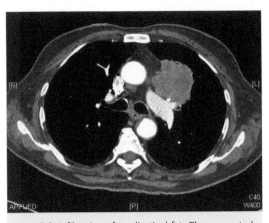

Fig. 15.2 Infiltration of mediastinal fat. The computed tomography (CT) shows an infiltration of mediastinal fat; therefore, the tumor is classified as T4 irrespective of its size.

singular (M1b) and multiple extrathoracic (M1c) metastases should be made.
• For optimal diagnostic quality, the study should be performed with contrast agent.

References

[1] El-Sherief AH, Lau CT, Wu CC, Drake RL, Abbott GF, Rice TW. International Association for the Study of Lung Cancer (IASLC) lymph node map: radiologic review with CT illustration. Radiographics. 2014; 34(6):1680–1691

[2] Detterbeck FC, Boffa DJ, Kim AW, Tanoue LT. The edition lung cancer stage classification. Chest. 2017; 151(1):193–203

[3] Ridge CA, Huang J, Cardoza S, et al. Comparison of multiplanar reformatted CT lung tumor measurements to axial tumor measurement alone: impact on maximal tumor dimension and T stage. AJR Am J Roentgenol. 2013; 201 (5):959–963

[4] Betancourt-Cuellar SL, Carter BW, Palacio D, Erasmus JJ. Pitfalls and limitations in non-small cell lung cancer staging. Semin Roentgenol. 2015; 50(3):175–182

16 Thyroid Ultrasound

Benjamin Wildman-Tobriner and Jenny K. Hoang

16.1 Template

Right lobe:

The right thyroid lobe [subjective description]. The right lobe measures [A × B × C] cm
Nodules as follows:
Nodule # [1/2/3/4]:

- Maximum size: [ ] cm; other 2 dimensions: [ ] cm
- Location: [upper/mid/lower]
- Composition: [cystic or almost completely cystic (0)/spongiform (0)/mixed cystic and solid (1)/solid/almost completely solid (2)/cannot determine (2)]
- Echogenicity: [anechoic (0)/hyperechoic (1)/isoechoic (1)/hypoechoic (2)/very hypoechoic (3)/cannot determine (1)]
- Shape: [not taller-than-wide (0)/taller-than-wide (3)]
- Margins: [smooth (0)/ill-defined (0)/lobulated or irregular (2)/extra-thyroidal extension (3)/cannot determine (0)]
- Echogenic foci: [none (0)/large comet-tail artifacts (0)/macrocalcifications (1)/peripheral calcifications (2)/punctate echogenic foci (3)]
- Additional echogenic foci 1: [large comet-tail artifacts (0)/macrocalcifications (1)/peripheral calcifications (2)/punctate echogenic foci (3)]
- Additional echogenic foci 2: [large comet-tail artifacts (0)/macrocalcifications (1)/peripheral calcifications (2)/punctate echogenic foci (3)]
- ACR TI-RADS total points: [ ]
- ACR TI-RADS risk category: [TR1 (0 points)/TR2 (2 points)/TR3 (3 points)/TR4 (4–6 points)/TR5 (≥ 7 points)]
- ACR TI-RADS recommendation: [ultrasound-guided fine needle aspiration/follow-up ultrasound in 1 year/no further follow-up]

If previously documented:

- Significant change in size (≥ 20% in two dimensions and minimal increase of 2 mm): [no/yes]
- Change in features: [no/yes]
- Change in ACR TI-RADS risk category: [no/yes]

Left lobe:

The left thyroid lobe [subjective description]. The left lobe measures [A × B × C] cm
- Repeat nodule template as above, if needed

Isthmus:

The isthmus [subjective description]
- Repeat nodule template as above, if needed

Impression:

- Summary of nodules that meet criteria for FNA
- Summary of nodules that meet criteria for follow-up imaging

16.2 Stakeholders

Endocrinologists, endocrinology surgeons, radiologists, and primary care physicians.

16.3 Pearls

- Thyroid nodules are often discovered incidentally on computed tomography (CT) and magnetic resonance imaging (MRI). We do not use structured reporting for these modalities but we do use cutoffs for when to recommend an ultrasound for further work-up of an incidental thyroid nodule:[1]
  - ≥ 1 cm in age less than 35.
  - ≥ 1.5 cm in age 35 or more.
- Using a structured report can increase report quality and improve consistency of giving management recommendations, with one study demonstrating a nearly 30% reduction in reports without a management recommendation.[2]
- Multiple societies have published guidelines for the work-up of thyroid nodules on ultrasound. Our practice uses the American College of Radiology Thyroid Imaging Reporting & Data System (ACR TI-RADS). ACR TI-RADS has been shown to improve specificity and reduce the number of unnecessary thyroid fine-needle aspirations (FNAs), with one study showing a 24% increase in specificity across readers.[3]
- Like many guidelines, ACR TI-RADS uses ultrasound features to assign risk to a nodule. There are five categories of features within ACR TI-RADS: composition, echogenicity, shape, margin, and echogenic foci. More than one type of echogenic focus can be assigned to a given nodule (▶ Fig. 16.1).

- One composition feature can be chosen, with solid or almost completely solid nodules conferring the highest risk (two points). A nodule should be ≥ 95% solid to be considered almost completely solid.
- One echogenicity features can be chosen. Very hypoechoic, the highest risk feature, is determined by comparing the echogenicity of the nodule to the overlying strap muscle. Nodules must be more hypoechoic than the muscle to be called very hypoechoic.
- Shape only has two options, with taller-than-wide nodules having higher risk. Taller-than-wide is determined subjectively in the transverse plane and should not be based on caliper measurements, as these may measure more oblique directions (▶ Fig. 16.2).
- Punctate echogenic foci can be difficult to discern. Comparison to background thyroid echogenicity is important to avoid overcalling this feature, as scanner type, scan settings, and background heterogeneity can make tissue "speckled" in appearance (both within and outside of nodules).
- Trying to standardize the way a practice interprets features can be beneficial. Division meetings with consensus reading of multiple cases can be helpful for establishing practice baselines.
- ACR TI-RADS calls for only the four most suspicious nodules to be followed. Consequently, sonographers at the point of care may be making decisions on what nodules to fully document

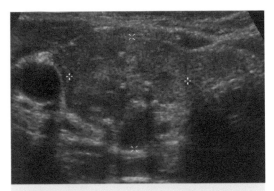

Fig. 16.1 Multiple types of echogenic foci can be assigned to a nodule. This nodule has shadowing macrocalcifications as well as scattered punctate echogenic foci.

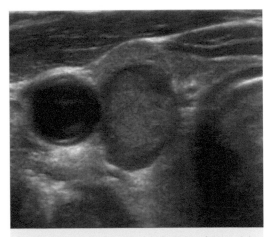

Fig. 16.2 Transverse ultrasound of a hypoechoic nodule that is taller-than-wide. The taller-than-wide shape suggests a nodule is growing against tissue planes and confers a higher risk.

and record. Sonographer education regarding the system is critical and allows for smoother workflow.

- ACR TI-RADS is detailed; maximizing the degree of template automation within dictation software can improve speed. Quick button "thumbing" across the template and pick-lists can facilitate reporting.

- Customized software may allow for automated point summation and easier recommendation field fill-in.[4] Natural language processing and machine learning will be able to assist with development of automated and facile templates.

- Communication with referring clinicians is critical; they have to be familiar with and approve of whatever guidelines a practice is using.

References

[1] Hoang JK, Langer JE, Middleton WD, et al. Managing incidental thyroid nodules detected on imaging: white paper of the ACR Incidental Thyroid Findings Committee. J Am Coll Radiol. 2015; 12(2):143–150

[2] Griffin AS, Mitsky J, Rawal U, Bronner AJ, Tessler FN, Hoang JK. Improved quality of thyroid ultrasound reports after implementation of the ACR thyroid imaging reporting and data system nodule lexicon and risk stratification system. J Am Coll Radiol. 2018; 15(5):743–748

[3] Hoang JK, Middleton WD, Farjat AE, et al. Reduction in thyroid nodule biopsies and improved accuracy with American College of Radiology thyroid imaging reporting and data system. Radiology. 2018; 287(1):185–193

[4] Wildman-Tobriner B, Ngo L, Jaffe TA, Ehieli WL, Ho LM, Lerebours R, Luo S, Allen BC. Automated structured reporting for thyroid ultrasound: effect on reporting errors and efficiency. J Am Coll Radiol. 2020 Aug 18:S1546-1440(20)30784-5.Epub ahead of print

Section III

Structured Reports in Abdominal Imaging

Editor: Olga R. Brook

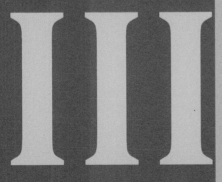

III

17 CT Colonography

Francesca Coppola and Judy Yee

17.1 Template

Indication:
- [Screening [asymptomatic, average/moderate risk]/
- Surveillance [asymptomatic, high risk]/
- Diagnostic examination in symptomatic patient [abdominal pain, diarrhea, constipation, gastrointestinal bleeding, anemia, intestinal obstruction, weight loss]/
- Following incomplete colonoscopy/
- Unable to undergo colonoscopy/
- Follow-up in patient with a colonic stoma or after colectomy/
- Prior to laparoscopic surgery for colorectal cancer][1]

Technique:
Preparation technique:
- Laxative: [PEG/magnesium citrate/sodium phosphate]
- Tagging regimen: [iodinated contrast media [..] mL/barium [..] mL/none]
- Spasmolytics: [none/hyoscine-N-butylbromide/glucagon]
- Insufflation: [manual/electronic] [air/CO2]
- Positions: [supine and prone/supine, prone and decubitus/right and left decubitus]
- Intravenous contrast media: [no/yes [ ] mL]
- Adverse events: [none/angina/arrhythmia/hypertension/hypotension/perforation/bleeding/other]

Visibility of the colonic mucosa: [complete/incomplete due to fecal residue in cecum/ascending/transverse/descending/sigmoid/rectum/incomplete due to suboptimal distention of cecum/ascending/transverse/descending/sigmoid/rectum][2]

Findings:
Colonic anatomy: [normal, abnormal] (specify abnormality).
Colonic abnormalities: [benign strictures/diverticula/extrinsic compression, ...]
Colonic lesion (specify for each lesion):
- Shape: [sessile/pedunculated/flat]
- Attenuation: [soft tissue/fat]
- Maximum diameter: [ ] mm, (polyps ≥ 6 mm are reported)
- Location: [cecum/ascending colon/transverse colon/descending colon/sigmoid colon/rectum]

Colonic mass (specify for each lesion):
- Shape: [annular, semiannular, vegetating)
- Maximum diameter: [ ] mm
- Location: [cecum/ascending colon/transverse colon/descending colon/sigmoid colon/rectum]

Extracolonic finding (specify for each):
- [size, location, lesion features]
- [anatomic variant/clinically unimportant/likely unimportant finding, incompletely evaluated/potentially important finding]

Conclusion:
Summary of lesions: [normal colon/benign lesions/indeterminate polyp/likely malignant lesions]
Extracolonic lesion: [absent/anatomic variant/clinically unimportant/likely unimportant finding, incompletely evaluated/potentially important finding]
Recommendation on follow-up: [routine screening/surveillance/colonoscopy/surgical referral]

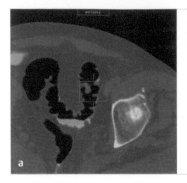
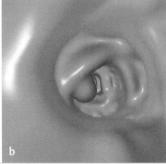

Fig. 17.1 Pedunculated sigmoid polyp: **(a)** 2D axial view, **(b)** 3D endoluminal view.

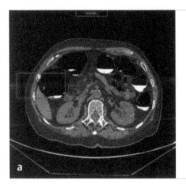
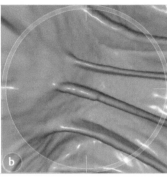

Fig. 17.2 Flat polyp: **(a)** 2D axial view, **(b)** 3D endoluminal view.

17.2 Stakeholders

Abdominal radiologists, gastroenterologists, and colorectal surgeons.

17.3 Pearls

- Any colonic segment that cannot be adequately evaluated for technical reasons should be documented. Size measurement of a polyp should be based on the largest diameter of the polyp head (excluding stalk, if present, of a pedunculated polyp) or at the base of a sessile polyp (▶ Fig. 17.1 and ▶ Fig. 17.2).
- In patients with only diminutive polyps ≤ 5 mm, the risk of high-grade dysplasia or cancer is extremely low. Reporting of these polyps is not recommended.
- All polyps 6 mm or larger should be reported.
- Extracolonic findings should be reported, taking into account the limitations of an unenhanced and/or low-dose technique used. A balanced approach for recommending further work-up of extracolonic findings is needed and should

consider the likelihood of a clinically important finding against the cost, patient anxiety, and possible complications due to additional evaluation.

- Most extracolonic findings are not clinically significant in screening cohorts. The rate of indeterminate or potentially relevant extracolonic findings (i.e., E3 or E4) in healthy adults ranges between 8 and 13%.[3]
- Usage of a computed tomography colonography (CTC) template results in higher reproducibility in comparison with use of a standard report with the possibility to adhere to validated classifications and guidelines,[4] with better interaction between radiologists and referring clinicians and the option to add key images and other metadata to the report.
- Use of the CT Colonography Reporting and Data System (C-RADS), which is a consensus statement of a standardized reporting structure for CTC findings, is recommended. Colorectal findings are categorized as C0 through C4 (▶ Table 17.1). Extracolonic findings are categorized as E0 through E4 (▶ Table 17.2).

Table 17.1 CT colonography reporting and data system (C-RADS)

Class	Description	Recommendation
C0	**Inadequate study/awaiting comparisons with priors**	
	• Inadequate prep; cannot exclude lesions ≥ 10 mm due to presence of fluid or feces	
	• Inadequate insufflation with one or more colonic segments collapsed on both views	
	• Awaiting prior studies for comparison	
C1	**Normal colon or benign lesion**	Continue routine screening
	• No visible abnormalities of the colon	
	• No polyp ≥ 6 mm	
	• Lipoma or inverted diverticulum	
	• Non-neoplastic findings (e.g., diverticulosis)	
C2	**Intermediate polyp or indeterminate finding**	Surveillance or colonoscopy
	• Intermediate polyp 6–9 mm, less than 3 in number	
	• Indeterminate findings, cannot exclude polyp ≥ 6 mm in technically adequate exam	
C3	**Polyp, possibly advanced adenoma**	Follow-up colonoscopy
	• Polyp ≥ 10 mm	
	• ≥ 3 polyps of 6–9 mm in size	
C4	**Colonic mass, likely malignant**	Surgical consult
	• Lesion compromises bowel lumen, with extracolonic invasion	

Source: Adapted from Zalis et al (2005).[5]

Table 17.2 Classifications of extracolonic findings

Class	Description	Recommendation
E0	**Limited exam**	
	• Study compromised by artifact; evaluation of extracolonic soft tissue is severely limited	
E1	**Normal exam or anatomical variant**	None
	No extracolonic findings	
	• Anatomical variant: double IVC	
E2	**Clinically unimportant finding**	No work-up is indicated
	• Liver, kidney: simple cysts	
	• Gallbladder: cholelithiasis	
	• Vertebra: hemangioma	
E3	**Likely unimportant finding, incompletely characterized**	Work-up may be indicated, based on patient preference and local practice
	• Minimally complex kidney cyst	
E4	**Potentially important finding**	Communicate with referring physician
	• Solid renal mass	
	• Lymphadenopathy	
	• Abdominal aortic aneurysm	
	• Noncalcified parenchymal pulmonary nodule ≥ 10 mm	

Source: Adapted from Zalis et al (2005).[5]

References

[1] Spada C, Stoker J, Alarcon O, et al. Clinical indications for computed tomographic colonography: European Society of Gastrointestinal Endoscopy (ESGE) and European Society of Gastrointestinal and Abdominal Radiology (ESGAR) Guideline. Eur Radiol. 2015; 25(2):331–345

[2] ACR–SAR–SCBT–MR Practice parameter for the performance of CT colonography in adults. https://www.acr.org/-/media/ACR/Files/Practice-Parameters/CT-Colonog.pdf?la=en. Accessed May 18, 2019

[3] Yee J, Chang KJ, Dachman AH, et al. The added value of the CT colonography reporting and data system (C-RADS). J Am Coll Radiol. 2016; 13(8):931–935

[4] Dachman AH, Barish MA. Structured reporting and quality control in CT colonography. Abdom Radiol (NY). 2018; 43 (3):566–573

[5] Zalis ME, Barish MA, Choi JR, et al. Working Group on Virtual Colonoscopy. CT colonography reporting and data system (C-RADS): a consensus statement. Radiology. 2005; 236(1):3–9

18 CT/MR Enterography

Benjamin Wildman-Tobriner

18.1 Template

Gastrointestinal:
Evidence of prior surgery: [ ]
Sites of involvement:
Stomach: [ ]
Small bowel:
- Disease location: [terminal ileum, jejunum, etc]
- Enhancement pattern and wall thickening: [mural stratification, homogeneous, thick, yes/no]
- Length of disease: [in cm]
- Edema and restricted diffusion (MRI only): [if yes, location]
- Stricture: [present, luminal narrowing without upstream dilatation, none]

Colon:
- Disease location: [ascending, transverse, etc.]
- Enhancement pattern and wall thickening: [mural stratification, homogeneous]
- Length of disease: [in cm]

Penetrating disease:
- Sinus tract: [if present, location]
- Fistula: [if present, location, what is connected to what]

Presence of steatorrhea: [present/absent]

Extraintestinal:
Mesenteric findings:
- Vasa recta: [engorged, normal]
- Mesenteric adenopathy: [present/absent]
- Fibrofatty proliferation: [present/absent]

Fluid collections: [if present, size and location, whether connected to fistula]
Perianal disease: [if present, can try to characterize on MRE]

Abdomen and pelvis: [remainder of organs]

Lower chest: [ ]

Musculoskeletal (MSK):

Sacroiliitis: [ ]

Avascular necrosis: [ ]

18.2 Stakeholders

Gastroenterologists and colorectal/general surgeons.

18.3 Pearls

- Both computed tomography (CT) and magnetic resonance (MR) enterography (CTE and MRE) have strong diagnostic performance for evaluation of inflammatory bowel disease (IBD) and its complications.
- Radiologists using structured reporting for CTE and MRE include more key disease features in their reports.[1]
- Referring clinicians have been shown to prefer structured reporting for IBD.[1]

- Though nonspecific, the most common feature of active Crohn disease is wall thickening, found in up to 82% of patients.[2]
- Hyperenhancement is also a common feature and can be seen as asymmetric, stratified, or homogeneous.
- In stratified enhancement, where both the inner wall and serosa are hyperenhancing, the innermost wall should not be referred to as "mucosal" hyperenhancement, as there may not be any viable mucosa at endoscopy. Rather, "inner wall" is a term that is increasingly used (▶ Fig. 18.1).
- The term "stricture" can be used when there is luminal narrowing of a small bowel loop and upstream dilatation greater than 3 cm. If the enlargement is less than 3 cm, the phrase "luminal narrowing without upstream dilatation" may be used.
- Radiologists should try to identify whether strictures are purely fibrotic or if they have an active inflammatory component, as the presence or absence of inflammation can influence management. For example, balloon dilatation is typically attempted on fibrotic strictures.
- Strictures and fistulas may occur simultaneously and in close proximity. Visualization of one entity should prompt evaluation for the other.[3,4]
- Small fluid collections and interloop abscesses can be difficult to detect (▶ Fig. 18.2). Having a high index of suspicion in this population as well as being prompted to look by a structured report can improve sensitivity for detection.
- Though they can be difficult to identify, ulcerations (breaks in the inner wall) have been shown to correlate with severe disease activity.[5]
- On MRE, mural edema as evidenced by increased T2 signal and diffusion restriction are also thought to correlate with more severe disease activity.
- Steatorrhea (▶ Fig. 18.3) is included in the template because its symptoms can mimic those of active IBD. Steatorrhea can occur in patients who have had extensive small bowel resection.
- Small field of view pelvic MRI can be used to provide good anatomic detail to evaluate perianal disease. If added to an imaging protocol, additional details can be added to the template.
- Templates should be customized based on referring clinician preference. For example, template items related to extraintestinal manifestations can be added or removed. Our institutional template does not include the

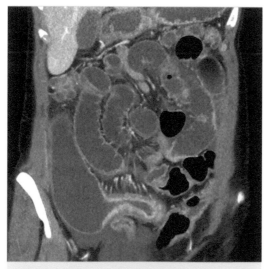

Fig. 18.1 Contrast-enhanced coronal computed tomography (CT). Marked wall thickening and inner wall hyperenhancement in the ileum of a patient with Crohn disease. Upstream dilatation of the ileum to more than 3 cm suggests a stricture with active inflammation. The inner wall may be devoid of a true mucosa at endoscopy, and thus the term "inner wall" is favored over "mucosa."

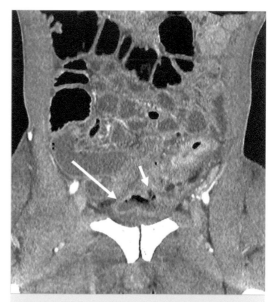

Fig. 18.2 Contrast-enhanced axial computed tomography (CT). Small pelvic abscess (*long arrow*) and a partially visualized fistula (*short arrow*) in a patient with active Crohn disease. These air and fluid containing collections can have a similar appearance to surrounding bowel and can be difficult to detect.

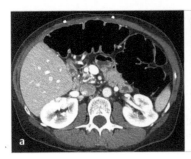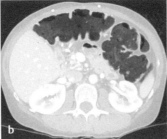

Fig. 18.3 (a, b) Contrast-enhanced axial CT of the same slice (soft tissue and lung windows) demonstrating steatorrhea. Apparent air-filled colon on soft tissue window is filled with low-density stool when viewed on a lung window. Steatorrhea can cause diarrhea that can mimic Crohn disease, so it is included in our template.

gallbladder, biliary tree, or renal stones, though these items (and others) can be considered.

- Quantitative scoring systems can be used to evaluate therapeutic response but are separate entities from structured reporting. Systems currently in use include the magnetic resonance index of activity (MaRIA) score or the Crohn disease MRI index (CDMI). The clinical utility of these systems remains an active area of research.

References

[1] Wildman-Tobriner B, Allen BC, Bashir MR, et al. Structured reporting of CT enterography for inflammatory bowel disease: effect on key feature reporting, accuracy across training levels, and subjective assessment of disease by referring physicians. Abdom Radiol (NY). 2017; 42(9):2243–2250

[2] Kim AY. Role of computed tomography enterography/magnetic resonance enterography: is it in prime time? Clin Endosc. 2012; 45(3):269–273

[3] Kelly JK, Preshaw RM. Origin of fistulas in Crohn's disease. J Clin Gastroenterol. 1989; 11(2):193–196

[4] Oberhuber G, Stangl PC, Vogelsang H, Schober E, Herbst F, Gasche C. Significant association of strictures and internal fistula formation in Crohn's disease. Virchows Arch. 2000; 437(3):293–297

[5] Bruining DH, Zimmermann EM, Loftus EV, Jr, Sandborn WJ, Sauer CG, Strong SA, Society of Abdominal Radiology Crohn's Disease-Focused Panel. Consensus recommendations for evaluation, interpretation, and utilization of computed tomography and magnetic resonance enterography in patients with small bowel Crohn's disease. Radiology. 2018; 286(3):776–799

19 Perianal Fistulizing Disease on MRI

Alejandro Garces-Descovich and Koenraad J. Mortele

19.1 Template

Internal anal opening:

Number of fistula openings
If multiple fistulas are found, please describe each one individually following the same template
No: _____

Fistula internal anal opening location
Please note position accordingly to quadrant and clock face location (supine)

☐ Anterior (midline)   ☐ Posterior (midline)

☐ Left anterolateral   ☐ Right anterolateral

☐ Left posterolateral   ☐ Right posterolateral

(1–12 o'clock)

Distance between internal anal opening and the anal verge
In millimeters_____ mm

Fistula Tract:

Maximum tract diameter
In millimeters_____ mm

Fistula type

Please note according to *Park's* classification for perianal fistulas

☐ Intersphincteric   ☐ Transphincteric   ☐ Extrasphincteric   ☐ Suprasphincteric   ☐ Superficial

Presence of secondary branches
Please note accordingly. If present, please describe where the branch extends

☐ None   ☐ One   ☐ Multiple   ☐ Extension:_____

Exit site location
Please note accordingly. Please circle the laterality as: left (L) or right (R)

☐ Gluteal   ☐ Scrotal   ☐ Vaginal   ☐ Labial   ☐ Urethral   ☐ Blind ending (sinus tract)
Left/Right   Left/Right   Left/Right   Left/Right   Left/Right   Left/Right

Hyperintensity of the tract on T2-weighted sequence (Van Assche classification)

☐ Absent   ☐ Mild   ☐ Marked

Enhancement of the fistula tract

☐ No central enhancement   ☐ Central enhancement with high-signal   ☐ Minimal progressive enhancement
(tract is fluid-filled)   intensity on T2 (granulation tissue)   with low-signal intensity on T2 (fibrosis)

Other findings:

Presence of abscess   ☐ YES ☐ NO

If "YES," please describe if the abscess is separated from the fistula tract, location, and size

☐ Separated ☐ Connected   Location: _____   Size: _____ mm

Please note if there is any of these specific additional findings:

☐ Anovaginal fistula   ☐ Rectal or sigmoid wall inflammation   ☐ Seton/drains/prior surgeries

19.2 Stakeholders

Colorectal surgeons, abdominal radiologists, gastroenterologists, and primary care physicians.

19.3 Pearls

- A structured reporting template for magnetic resonance imaging (MRI) in patients with perianal fistulizing disease misses fewer key features for surgical treatment than narrative reports.[1]
- A perianal fistulizing disease MRI reporting template missed 0.3 ± 0.9 (range 1–5) out of 12 key features, as compared to narrative reports that missed 6.3 ± 1.8 (range 3–11) key features for surgical planning of perianal fistulas.
- Implementation of a structured reporting template for MRI in patients with perianal fistulizing disease has been described to be more complete and clearer to understand.
- Perianal fistula classifications are helpful for management. One can use Park's classification (used for surgical planning) (▶ Fig. 19.1), Van Assche classification, and/or St. James University Hospital classification (MRI-based grading systems) (▶ Fig. 19.2) (▶ Table 19.1).
- The MRI report should mention the number of fistulas, as a bigger number relates to more challenging treatment and a higher number of surgical and postsurgical complications.
- Assessment of the distance between the internal anal opening (IAO) and the anal verge, as well as the relation between IAO and internal anal sphincter, is necessary, as it aids with surgical preparation (▶ Fig. 19.3 and ▶ Fig. 19.4).
- Reporting of secondary tracks is needed, as they may be complicated by abscess formation and might require specific surgical techniques to ensure proper drainage.
- Hyperintensity on T2, along with assessment of contrast enhancement of the tract, is vital, as according to the Van Assche classification it defines fistula activity.[2]
- Notification of drainage catheters, setons, and features of prior surgical history is helpful, as they estimate the rate of success of prior management (▶ Fig. 19.5).[3]

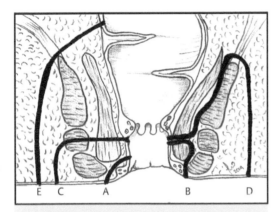

Fig. 19.1 Anatomical types of fistulas based on relation to the internal and external sphincters according to Park's classification. A, superficial; B, intersphincteric; C, transphincteric; D, suprasphincteric; E, extrasphincteric. (Adapted from Parks et al 1976[4].)

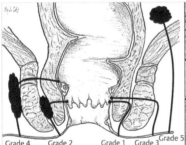 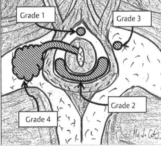

Fig. 19.2 Types of fistula based on anatomic landmarks in the axial plane according to St. James University Hospital classification. (Adapted from de Miguel Criado et al 2012.[5])

Table 19.1 Magnetic resonance-based grading systems

Van Assche MRI severity score for perianal Crohn disease[a]

Used by radiologist as a reference at follow-up imaging to assess improvement or worsening of fistula activity

Number of fistula tracts	Score
• None	0
• Single, unbranched	1
• Single, branched	2
• Multiple	3
Location	
• Extra- or intersphincteric	1
• Transphincteric	2
• Suprasphincteric	3
Extension	
• Infralevatoric	1
• Supralevatoric	2
Hyperintensity on T2-weighted images	
• Absent	0
• Mild	4
• Pronounced	8
Collections (cavities greater than 3 cm in diameter)	
• Absent	0
• Present	4
Rectal wall involvement	
• Normal	0
• Thickened	2
St. James University Hospital classification[b]	
Based on anatomic landmarks in the **axial** plane	
Grade 1	Simple linear intersphincteric
Grade 2	Intersphincteric with abscess or secondary tract
Grade 3	Simple linear transphincteric
Grade 4	Transphincteric with abscess or secondary tract in ischiorectal or ischioanal fossa
Grade 5	Supralevator and translevator extension

[a]Adapted from Van Assche et al 2003.[2]
[b]Adapted from de Miguel Criado et al 2012.[5]

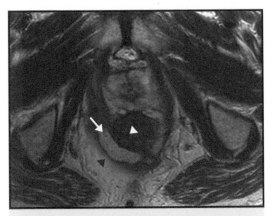

Fig. 19.3 Axial T2-weighted image show presence of an intersphincteric fistula (*arrow*) between the internal sphincter (*white arrowhead*) and external sphincter (*black arrowhead*).

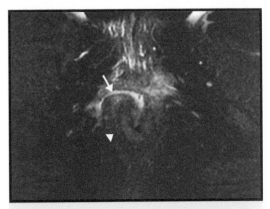

Fig. 19.4 Axial T2-weighted image show presence of a transphincteric fistula (*arrow*) traversing the internal sphincter (*black arrowhead*) and external sphincter (*white arrowhead*).

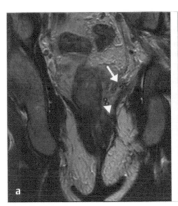

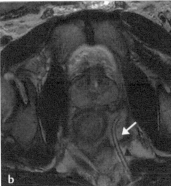

Fig. 19.5 (a, b) Coronal T2- and axial T2-weighted images show presence of a percutaneous catheter drainage (*arrowheads*) allowing drainage of a suprasphincteric (*arrow*) abscess.

References

[1] Tuncyurek O, Garces-Descovich A, Jaramillo-Cardoso A, et al. Structured versus narrative reporting of pelvic MRI in perianal fistulizing disease: impact on clarity, completeness, and surgical planning. Abdom Radiol (NY). 2019;44(3):811–820. doi: 10.1007/s00261-018-1858-8

[2] Van Assche G, Vanbeckevoort D, Bielen D, et al. Magnetic resonance imaging of the effects of infliximab on perianal fistulizing Crohn's disease. Am J Gastroenterol. 2003; 98 (2):332–339

[3] Ong EM, Ghazi LJ, Schwartz DA, Mortelé KJ, Crohn's & Colitis Foundation of America, Inc. Guidelines for imaging of Crohn's perianal fistulizing disease. Inflamm Bowel Dis. 2015; 21 (4):731–736

[4] Parks AG, Gordon PH, Hardcastle JD. A classification of fistula-in-ano. Br J Surg. 1976; 63(1):1–12

[5] de Miguel Criado J, del Salto LG, Rivas PF, et al. MR imaging evaluation of perianal fistulas: spectrum of imaging features. Radiographics. 2012; 32(1):175–194

20 Adrenal Incidentaloma on CT/MRI

Tarik K. Alkasab, Bernardo C. Bizzo, and Renata Rocha de Almeida Bizzo

20.1 Template

History of malignancy: [known/no/unknown]
Findings:
- There is a [ ] cm × [ ] cm lesion in the [lateral limb/medial limb/body] of the [right/left] adrenal gland
- The contralateral adrenal gland is [normal/thickened without discrete nodule]

Unenhanced computed tomography (CT) scan:
The lesion has attenuation of [less than −20/less than or equal to 10/between 10 and 50/equal or greater than 50] HU, [homogeneous/heterogenous] density with [diffuse/partial/punctate/dysmorphic/coarse/irregular/curvilinear/no] calcifications, and [well-defined/blurred] margins.

Enhanced (60–90 s) and delayed (15 min) CT scan:
The lesion has [fluid/greater than 20 HU/fat] attenuation with [diffuse/partial/punctate/dysmorphic/coarse/irregular/curvilinear/no] calcifications, [well-defined/blurred] margins, and shows [homogeneous/heterogenous] enhancement in the portal venous phase.
The lesion demonstrates [less than 40%/equal or greater than 40%] relative washout of contrast.

Adrenal CT protocol: Unenhanced, enhanced (60–90 s), and delayed (15 min) CT scan:
The lesion has attenuation of [less than −20/less than or equal to 10/between 10 and 50/equal or greater than 50] HU with [diffuse/partial/punctate/dysmorphic/coarse/irregular/curvilinear/no] calcifications on unenhanced CT phase and shows [no/heterogeneous/homogeneous] enhancement in the portal venous phase.
The lesion demonstrates [less than 60%/equal or greater than 60%] absolute washout of contrast.

Magnetic resonance imaging (MRI):
The lesion shows signal [hyper/hypo] intensity on T1-weighted images and signal [hyper/hypo] intensity on T2-weighted images.
The lesion [demonstrates/does not demonstrate] loss of signal on opposed-phase compared to in-phase imaging and [shows/does not show] signal dropout on fat-suppressed MRI sequences.
The lesion has [no/heterogeneous/homogeneous] enhancement.

Impression/Recommendation:
[Left/Right] adrenal lesion has benign diagnostic features in keeping with an adrenal [myelolipoma/hematoma/cyst/sequelae of old granulomatous disease]. No additional work-up is recommended.
[Left/Right] adrenal lesion has microscopic fat likely representing a lipid-rich benign adenoma. No additional imaging work-up is recommended. Endocrine screening is advised as lipid-rich adenomas may be hormonally active with subclinical features.
[Left/Right] adrenal lesion shows washout characteristics of a lipid-poor benign adenoma. No additional imaging work-up is recommended. Endocrine screening is advised as lipid-poor adenomas may be hormonally active with subclinical features.
Indeterminate [left/right] adrenal lesion due to lack of benign washout characteristics. In a patient without a history of cancer, consider 6/12-month follow-up CT to document stability, biopsy, or resection. Endocrine screening is advised, as indeterminate lesions may be hormonally active with subclinical features. In a patient with a known history of cancer, consider PET-CT or biopsy for further lesion characterization with prior endocrine screening to determine functional status and exclude pheochromocytoma.
Large/necrotic/heterogenous [left/right] adrenal lesion. Consider surgical resection with prior endocrine screening to determine functional status and exclude pheochromocytoma.

20.2 Stakeholders

Endocrinologists, gastroenterologists, and abdominal and interventional radiologists.

20.3 Pearls

- History of malignancy has implications on recommendations for the work-up of adrenal incidentalomas according to the American College of Radiology (ACR) White Paper on the Management of Incidental Adrenal Masses (▶ Table 20.1).[1]
- Lesions containing macroscopic fat (less than – 20 Hounsfield unit [HU] on unenhanced computed tomography (CT) or low signal on fat-suppressed magnetic resonance imaging (MRI) images) are most likely myelolipomas which do not require additional work-up, or rarely adrenal adenomas, adrenocortical carcinomas, pheochromocytomas, liposarcomas, or collision tumors.[1,2]
- Lesions with microscopic fat (less than or equal to 10 HU on unenhanced CT (▶ Fig. 20.1) or signal dropout on opposed phase compared to in-phase MRI images) are most likely to represent lipid-rich adenomas, which do not

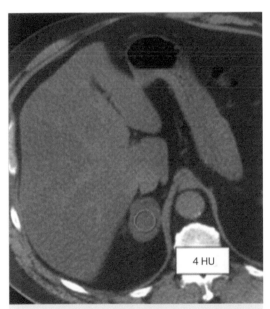

Fig. 20.1 Right adrenal lesion with well-defined margins and attenuation of 4 Hounsfield unit (HU) (≤ 10 HU) on unenhanced computed tomography (CT) due to microscopic fat content likely representing a lipid-rich adenoma.

require further imaging work-up, or rarely adrenocortical carcinomas and metastases from hepatocellular or renal cell carcinomas. Virtual noncontrast and water density images from dual-energy CT can also be used to characterize lipid-rich adenomas using the ≤ 10 HU cutoff.
- Lesions without enhancement such as adrenal cysts and primary hemorrhage do not require additional work-up.[1,2] Attenuation of 50–90 HU on unenhanced CT is diagnostic of the acute stage of adrenal hemorrhage.[2]
- Normal-sized or atrophic gland containing benign calcifications (e.g., diffuse, bilateral, or coarse and irregular), such as old hematomas and sequelae of prior granulomatous disease, do not require further work-up.[2,3]
- Punctate, dystrophic, or peripheral curvilinear calcifications within an adrenal lesion are less specific and can be found in both benign (e.g., myelolipoma, hemangioma, and pseudocyst) and malignant entities (e.g., adrenocortical carcinomas, sarcomas, and metastases).[2,3]
- Lesions without benign diagnostic features (e.g., macroscopic fat, absent enhancement, diffuse and bilateral calcifications) or history of malignancy, and measuring ≥ 1 cm and < 4 cm are considered indeterminate and require further imaging and biochemical work-up.
- *Relative washout* of contrast (▶ Fig. 20.2) is calculated when the unenhanced CT is not available, using the formula: (portal venous [PV] enhanced HU – 15-min delayed HU)/PV enhanced HU × 100%. A value of ≥ 40% is diagnostic of a benign adenoma.[1]
- *Absolute washout* of contrast is calculated on the adrenal lesion CT protocol using the formula: (PV enhanced HU – 15-min delayed HU)/(PV enhanced HU – unenhanced HU) × 100%. A value of ≥ 60% is diagnostic of a benign lipid-poor adenoma. However, pheochromocytomas may rarely mimic benign adenomas by showing > 60% washout.[1]
- Avid PV enhancement (>110 HU) raises suspicion of pheochromocytomas.[1]
- Imaging findings such as size ≥ 4 cm, necrosis, heterogeneity, < 40% relative or < 60% absolute washout of contrast, no signal dropout on chemical selective MRI, and vascular invasion raise suspicion of neoplasms, including primary adrenal carcinoma, pheochromocytomas, or metastases in patients with known cancer.[2]
- A scoring system based on density (10% of HU), contour (+ 2 if blurred), homogeneity (+ 1 if

Table 20.1 American College of Radiology recommendations for the management of incidental adrenal lesions with templated work-up recommendations

Diagnostic benign imaging features	Cancer history	Size (cm)	Contrast wash-out	Template recommendations
Macroscopic fat Hematoma No enhancement Benign calcifications[a]	N/A	N/A	N/A	No additional work-up is recommended.
Microscopic fat	N/A	N/A	N/A	No additional imaging work-up is recommended. Endocrine screening is advised as lipid-rich adenomas may be hormonally active with subclinical features.
None	No or unknown	≥1–≤2	N/A	Consider follow-up adrenal CT protocol in 12 months. Endocrine screening is advised as indeterminate lesions may be hormonally active with subclinical features.
		>2–<4[b]	APW/RPW ≥60/40%	No additional imaging work-up is recommended. Endocrine screening is advised as lipid-poor adenomas may be hormonally active with subclinical features.
			APW/RPW <60/40%	Consider 6/12-month follow-up CT to document stability, biopsy, or resection. Endocrine screening is advised as indeterminate lesions may be hormonally active with subclinical features.
		≥4	N/A	Consider surgical resection with prior endocrine screening to determine functional status and exclude pheochromocytoma.
	Yes, without known metastases	≥1–<4[b]	APW/RPW ≥60/40%	No additional imaging work-up is recommended. Endocrine screening is advised as lipid-poor adenomas may be hormonally active with subclinical features.
			APW/RPW <60/40%	Consider PET-CT or biopsy with prior endocrine screening to determine functional status and exclude pheochromocytoma.
		≥4	N/A	Consider PET-CT or biopsy with prior endocrine screening to determine functional status and exclude pheochromocytoma.

Abbreviations: APW, absolute percentage washout; CT, computed tomography; PET-CT, positron emission tomography–computed tomography (PET-CT) RPW, relative percentage washout.
Source: Adapted from Mayo-Smith et al 2017.[1]
Note: Incidental lesion with short axis <1 cm need not be pursued.
[a]Normal-sized or atrophic gland containing diffuse, bilateral, or coarse and irregular calcifications, such as old hematomas and sequelae of prior granulomatous disease.
[b]If unenhanced CT only, template recommendations: Adrenal CT protocol is recommended for further characterization. As these lesions may be hormonally active with subclinical features, further evaluation for endocrine hyperfunction is advised.

heterogeneous), and size (cm) showed high accuracy to differentiate adenomas from metastases in patients with a known malignancy by using a seven-point threshold.[4]

• The presence of recommendations for the work-up of adrenal incidentalomas in the radiology report as well as the use of structured, templated, and standardized terminology

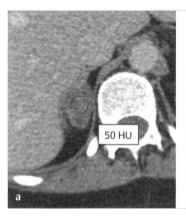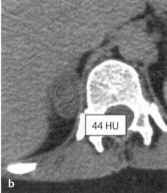

Fig. 20.2 Right adrenal lesion with attenuation of 50 Hounsfield unit (HU) on enhanced portal venous phase computed tomography (CT) **(a)** and 44 HU on 15-min delayed CT **(b)**. The calculated relative washout is 12% consistent with an indeterminate lesion.

(▶ Table 20.1) have shown to increase ordering provider compliance.[5,6]

References

[1] Mayo-Smith WW, Song JH, Boland GL, et al. Management of incidental adrenal masses: a white paper of the ACR Incidental Findings Committee. J Am Coll Radiol. 2017; 14(8):1038–1044

[2] Garrett RW, Nepute JC, Hayek ME, Albert SG. Adrenal incidentalomas: clinical controversies and modified recommendations. AJR Am J Roentgenol. 2016; 206(6):1170–1178

[3] Sargar KM, Khanna G, Hulett Bowling R. Imaging of nonmalignant adrenal lesions in children. Radiographics. 2017; 37(6):1648–1664

[4] Gufler H, Eichner G, Grossmann A, et al. Differentiation of adrenal adenomas from metastases with unenhanced computed tomography. J Comput Assist Tomogr. 2004; 28 (6):818–822

[5] Wickramarachchi BN, Meyer-Rochow GY, McAnulty K, Conaglen JV, Elston MS. Adherence to adrenal incidentaloma guidelines is influenced by radiology report recommendations. ANZ J Surg. 2016; 86(6):483–486

[6] Maher DI, Williams E, Grodski S, Serpell JW, Lee JC. Adrenal incidentaloma follow-up is influenced by patient, radiologic, and medical provider factors: a review of 804 cases. Surgery. 2018; 164(6):1360–1365

21 Ovarian and Adenxal Cysts on Ultrasound

Elizabeth V. Craig, Jeanne M. Horowitz, and Krupa K. Patel-Lippmann

21.1 Template

Adnexa:
- Lesion in the [right/left/midline] [ovary/adnexa] measures [ ] × [ ] × [ ] cm
- Loculations: [unilocular/multilocular]
- Solid components: [no/solitary/multiple (give number)]
- Maximal diameter of largest solid component: [ ] cm
- Doppler flow in solid component: [none/minimal/moderate/very strong]
- Cystic component: [anechoic/hyperechoic/homogenous low-level echoes/scattered low-level echoes/fluid-fluid level/reticular pattern]
- Internal cyst wall: [smooth/irregular/contains calcifications]
- Other: [no free fluid/anechoic fluid in the cul-de-sac/fluid containing echoes/ascites]

Uterus:
- Uterus: [anteverted/mid-positioned/retroverted] measuring [ ] × [ ] × [ ] cm
- Endometrium: [could not be identified/homogeneous/heterogeneous] measuring [ ] mm

21.2 Stakeholders

Gynecologists and primary care physicians.

21.3 Pearls

- Adnexal cysts are a common finding in the pre- and postmenopausal patient, with the vast majority of these lesions being benign.
- Most cysts in premenopausal females are of follicular origin and will resolve within one to two menstrual cycles.[1,2]
- Lesions demonstrating solid components or vascularity are more likely to be malignant.
- The goal of the radiologist is to triage adnexal cysts into those that are likely benign and those that are suspicious for neoplasm.
- The International Ovarian Tumor Analysis (IOTA) group published the first international lexicon for adnexal lesions in 2000 with the goal of standardizing reporting to improve diagnostic accuracy.[3]
- In 2018, the American College of Radiology (ACR) developed a lexicon utilizing evidence-based data from the IOTA group creating O-RADS (Ovarian-Adnexal Reporting and Data System).[4]
- The O-RADS terminology has been used in the provided template.
- Using O-RADS, adnexal cystic lesions can be broadly classified into one of four categories based on the number of locules (unilocular vs. multilocular) and solid elements (presence or absence) (▶ Fig. 21.1 and ▶ Fig. 21.2).
- A *solid component* (also called a "papillary projection") is present if it measures ≥ 3 mm; otherwise, this is considered irregularity of the cyst wall.
- The risk of malignancy increases when there are ≥ 4 papillary projections, or a solid, vascularized nodule.[5]
- Cyst wall thickening, clot, and the echogenic portions of a dermoid cyst are *not* considered solid components.
- *Clot* is avascular with angular margins, and it may move when external pressure is applied with the transvaginal US probe.

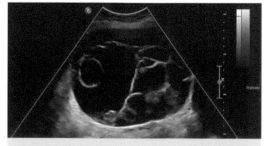

Fig. 21.1 This multilocular cyst contains anechoic fluid and several papillary projections, some of which demonstrate Doppler flow. This was resected with pathology revealing a borderline mucinous cystadenoma.

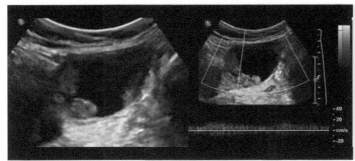

Fig. 21.2 A unilocular cyst demonstrates features which are suspicious for malignancy including more than four papillary projections (only three pictured) and Doppler flow within the solid components. Note: spectral Doppler shows a low resistance arterial waveform. This was a clear cell carcinoma arising from an endometriotic cyst.

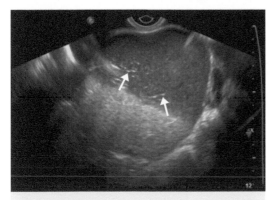

Fig. 21.3 Hyperechoic lines and dots (*arrows*) represent pieces of hair in this dermoid cyst.

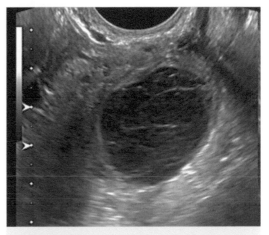

Fig. 21.4 Characteristic reticular pattern is seen in a hemorrhagic cyst.

- Internal Doppler flow (either color or power) is diagnostic of solid tissue and can be graded on a 1–4 scale (no flow, minimal, moderate, very strong); however, lack of flow does not necessarily exclude solid tissue.
- Adnexal lesions should be measured in three perpendicular planes. The number of solid components and size of the largest nodule should be recorded. Larger solid components may carry higher risk of malignancy.[4,5] Nodule contour may be reported as smooth or irregular. Internal cystic contents are described by echogenicity, presence of a fluid–fluid level or other characteristic descriptor.
- Some adnexal lesions have classic imaging features allowing for a confident diagnosis based on pattern recognition. These lesions include:
  - *Endometrioma*: Homogenous low-level echoes or "ground-glass" echotexture.
  - *Dermoid* (mature cystic teratoma): Echogenic component with posterior acoustic shadowing; hyperechoic lines and dots; floating echogenic spherical structures (▶ Fig. 21.3).
  - *Hemorrhagic cyst*: Reticular pattern of internal echoes and/or retracting clot (▶ Fig. 21.4).
  - *Hydrosalpinx*: Tubular structure with incomplete septations and/or endosalpingeal folds (small round projections on the inner walls giving the appearance of "beads on a string").
  - *Peritoneal inclusion cyst*: Usually a large cystic space immediately adjacent to or containing the ovary and conforming to the shape of the pelvis; often seen in patients with a history of surgery, endometriosis, or pelvic inflammation.

References

[1] Valentin L, Ameye L, Franchi D, et al. Risk of malignancy in unilocular cysts: a study of 1148 adnexal masses classified as unilocular cysts at transvaginal ultrasound and review of the literature. Ultrasound Obstet Gynecol. 2013; 41(1):80–89

[2] Levine D, Brown DL, Andreotti RF, et al. Management of asymptomatic ovarian and other adnexal cysts imaged at US:

Society of Radiologists in Ultrasound Consensus Conference statement. Radiology. 2010; 256(3):943–954

[3] Timmerman D, Valentin L, Bourne TH, Collins WP, Verrelst H, Vergote I, International Ovarian Tumor Analysis (IOTA) Group. Terms, definitions and measurements to describe the sonographic features of adnexal tumors: a consensus opinion from the International Ovarian Tumor Analysis (IOTA) Group. Ultrasound Obstet Gynecol. 2000; 16(5):500–505

[4] Andreotti RF, Timmerman D, Benacerraf BR, et al. Ovarian-adnexal reporting lexicon for ultrasound: a white paper of the ACR Ovarian-Adnexal Reporting and Data System Committee. J Am Coll Radiol. 2018; 15(10):1415–1429

[5] Timmerman D, Testa AC, Bourne T, et al. Simple ultrasound-based rules for the diagnosis of ovarian cancer. Ultrasound Obstet Gynecol. 2008; 31(6):681–690

22 Fibroid MRI

Olga R. Brook

22.1 Template

> **Uterus:**
> The uterus is [anteverted/mid-positioned/retroverted] measuring [ ] × [ ] × [ ] cm
> Endometrium: [could not be identified/homogeneous/heterogeneous] measuring [ ] mm
> Junctional zone: [ ] mm [without focal thickening/with focal thickening at ___]
> **Fibroids:**
> Fibroid burden: [none/(specify # between 1–5)/6–10/11–15/>15/too many to count]
> Fibroid enhancement: [none/homogenous/heterogenous]
> Submucosal fibroids (all submucosal fibroids are listed below):
>   1. None
>   2. Size [ ] × [ ] × [ ] cm, [location], with thinnest portion of overlying myometrium extending from fibroid to serosa measuring [ ] mm
>
> In addition, the three dominant fibroids are:
>   1. Size [ ] × [ ] × [ ] cm, [enhancement], [clinical type], [location]
>   2. Size [ ] × [ ] × [ ] cm, [enhancement], [clinical type], [location]
>   3. Size [ ] × [ ] × [ ] cm, [enhancement], [clinical type], [location]
>
> No evidence of cornual or cervical fibroids
> Vascular supply to the uterus: [uterine arteries/uterine and [right and left/right/left] ovarian arteries]
> **Ovaries:**
> [Normal ovarian size with normal follicular activity bilaterally/normal size without follicular activity]
> [no evidence of free fluid/physiological amount of free fluid]

22.2 Stakeholders

Minimally invasive gynecological surgeons and interventional radiologists.

22.3 Pearls

- Fibroid magnetic resonance imaging (MRI) templates have been shown to provide essential information for treatment planning for both minimally invasive gynecological surgeons and interventional radiologists.[1]
- Structured reports missed only 1.2 ± 1.5 out of 19 key features, as compared to narrative reports that missed 7.3 ± 2.5 key features for planning of fibroid treatment. Structured reports were more helpful and easier to understand by clinicians.
- Total uterine size should include the whole uterus with exophytic fibroids, as total uterine and fibroid dimensions are required for surgical planning (open vs. laparoscopic approach).
- Uterine size should also include cervix, per convention (► Fig. 22.1).
- Overlying myometrial thickness from the fibroid to the serosa is needed for submucosal fibroids, as this would direct whether hysteroscopic fibroid resection is feasible (► Fig. 22.2) without risk of uterine perforation.[2]
- Presence of cervical and cornual fibroids is important for myomectomy planning, as this location increases risk of significant bleeding, unplanned hysterectomy, and damage to the ureter and fallopian tube.[3]
- Fibroid classification is important to facilitate common language with referring physicians. One can use either FIGO classification (used mostly for research purposes) or clinical classification (► Table 22.1).[4]
- Adenomyosis (diagnosed with thickening of junctional zone greater than 12 mm) would require smaller size of embolization particles at the time of uterine artery embolization. In

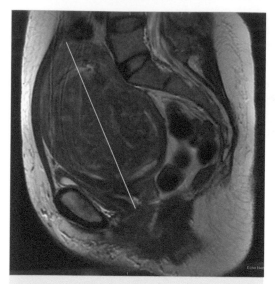

Fig. 22.1 Craniocaudal length of the uterus should include cervix, per convention.

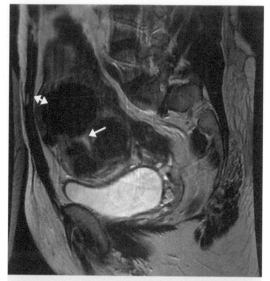

Fig. 22.2 Overlying myometrial thickness (*double arrow*) of submucosal fibroid is important to prevent perforation of the uterus during hysteroscopic myomectomy. *Arrow* denotes endometrial cavity.

addition, outcomes of uterine artery embolization for adenomyosis are slightly different as compared to uterine artery embolization for fibroids, which is important in patient counseling prior to the procedure.
- Enhancement of the fibroids determines whether patient is appropriate candidate for uterine artery embolization.
- Presence of collateral supply to the uterus and fibroids from ovarian arteries may impact uterine artery embolization planning

(transfemoral vs. transradial approach), in addition to being important in patient counseling prior to the procedure.
- Intracavitary and some submucosal fibroids may expel after uterine artery embolization, usually a few months postoperative. This possibility is important in preprocedural counseling.

Table 22.1 Fibroid classification

FIGO classification			Clinical classification	
		Description	Description	Clinical type
SM—Submucosal	0	Pedunculated intracavitary	Pedunculated submucosal = entirely cavitary with stalk attachment	Submucosal (FIGO 0–1)
			Cavitary submucosal (entirely cavitary with broad base attachment)	
	1	< 50% intramural	Submucosal with < 50% intramural component	
	2	≥ 50% intramural	Intramural with ≤ 50% submucosal component	Intramural (FIGO 2–5)
O—Other	3	Contacts endometrium, 100% intramural	Intramural, abutting endometrium	
	4	Intramural	100% Intramural = intramural without submucosal or subserosal component	
	5	Subserosal, ≥ 50% intramural	Intramural with ≤ 50% subserosal component	
	6	Subserosal, < 50% intramural	Subserosal with < 50% intramural component	Subserosal (FIGO 6–7)
	7	Subserosal pedunculated	Pedunculated subserosal (entirely exophytic with stalk attachment)	
			Exophytic subserosal (entirely subserosal fibroid with broad base attachment)	
	8	Other (e.g., cervical, parasitic)	Other (e.g., cervical, broad ligament, cornual, parasitic fibroids)	Other (FIGO 8)
Hybrid	Two numbers are listed separated by a hyphen. By convention, the first refers to the relationship with the endometrium, while the second refers to the relationship to the serosa. One example below:			Hybrid
	2–5	Submucosal and subserosal, each with less than half the diameters in the endometrial and peritoneal cavities, respectively.	Transmyometrial fibroid (e.g., spanning the entire myometrium) with submucosal and subserosal components	

Source: Adapted from Munro MG et al 2011.[4]

References

[1] Franconeri A, Fang J, Carney B, et al. Structured vs narrative reporting of pelvic MRI for fibroids: clarity and impact on treatment planning. Eur Radiol. 2018; 28(7):3009–3017

[2] Deshmukh SP, Gonsalves CF, Guglielmo FF, Mitchell DG. Role of MR imaging of uterine leiomyomas before and after embolization. Radiographics. 2012; 32(6):E251–E281. Review. PubMed PMID: 23065174

[3] McLucas B. Diagnosis, imaging and anatomical classification of uterine fibroids. Best Pract Res Clin Obstet Gynaecol. 2008; 22(4):627–642

[4] Munro MG, Critchley HO, Broder MS, Fraser IS, FIGO Working Group on Menstrual Disorders. FIGO classification system (PALM-COEIN) for causes of abnormal uterine bleeding in nongravid women of reproductive age. Int J Gynaecol Obstet. 2011; 113(1):3–13

23 Pelvic Floor Dysfunction

Victoria Chernyak

23.1 Template

Functional evaluation:
Patient [did/did not] defecate adequately during the examination
Pelvic floor function:
H line (levator hiatus):
- Rest: [ ] cm (normal ≤5 cm)
- Defection/maximal strain: [ ] cm

M line (anorectal junction location relative to PCL):
- Rest: [ ] cm [above/below] (normal ≤ 2 cm below)
- Defecation/maximal strain: [ ] cm [above/below]

The findings are consistent with [normal/widened] levator hiatus and [normal/low lying] anorectal junction at rest with [mild/moderate/severe] pelvic floor relaxation during [defecation/maximal strain]
Anorectal angle:
- Rest: [ ] degrees
- Kegel: [ ] degrees
- Defecation/maximal strain: [ ] degrees

The findings are consistent with [normal/narrowed/widened] resting angle [with/without] expected narrowing during Kegel and [expected widening/paradoxical contraction] during defecation/maximal strain
Anterior compartment:
Bladder base location relative to the [pubococcygeal line/midpubic line]:
- Rest: [ ] cm [above/below]
- Defecation/Maximal strain: [ ] cm [above/below]

The findings are consistent with [no/mild/moderate/severe] cystocele.
Urethral hypermobility: [present/absent]
Middle compartment:
[Vaginal apex/anterior cervical lip] location relative to [pubococcygeal line/midpubic line]:
- Rest: [ ] cm [above/below]
- Defecation/Maximal strain: [ ] cm [above/below]

The findings are consistent with [no/mild/moderate/severe] [uterine/vaginal] prolapse.
Cul-de-sac hernias: [none/peritoneocele/enterocele/sigmoidocele] [*specify the distance from the pubococcygeal line if present*]
Posterior compartment:
Anterior rectocele: [none/mild/moderate/severe] [*specify details if present*]
Rectal intussusception: [none/mucosal/full-thickness] [*if present, specify if intrarectal, intra-anal or extra-anal*]
Anatomic evaluation:
Levator muscles: [within normal limits/*describe relevant abnormalities*]
Internal anal sphincter muscle: [normal in thickness, length, and signal/(*describe abnormality*)]
External anal sphincter muscle: [normal in thickness, length, and signal/(*describe abnormality*)]
Other: [none/*describe relevant anatomic findings (e.g., urethral support ligaments) and pertinent surgical changes (e.g., hysterectomy, urethral slings, vaginal mesh, urethral bulking agent*]
Incidental findings: [none/*specify details if present*]

23.2 Stakeholders

Gynecologists, urogynecologists, urologists, gastroenterologists, and colorectal surgeons.

23.3 Pearls

- In the technique section, report whether the rectal and/or vaginal gel was administered, and describe the position of imaging (i.e., supine, upright, or other).
- Defecation is essential for accurate assessment of pelvic floor function and pelvic organ prolapse. Include in the report if the patient was unable to defecate during the examination, since then the results may underestimate the degree of pathology.[1]
- The report template should be tailored to the needs of the referring clinicians. For example, the reports of patients with constipation referred by gastroenterologists require an explicit statement on whether pelvic floor dyssynergia (PFD) is present or absent, whereas the reports of patients with urinary incontinence referred by urogynecologists may omit a statement that PFD is absent. Conversely, the detailed description of urethral support ligaments, whether normal or not, may be necessary for all patients referred by urogynecologists, but not for all patients referred by gastroenterologists. A discussion with the referrers helps ensuring that all the information relevant clinically is included in the report.
- The pubococcygeal line (PCL), H line, and M line assess presence/degree of pelvic floor relaxation (▶ Table 23.1 and ▶ Fig. 23.1).[2,3,4]
- The *PCL* represents the level of the pelvic floor, and is drawn from the most inferior aspect of the pubic symphysis to the last coccygeal joint.
- The *H line* represents anteroposterior length of the levator hiatus, and is drawn from the most inferior aspect of the pubic symphysis to the

posterior rectal wall at the level of the anorectal junction.
- The *M line* represents the degree of muscular pelvic floor descent, and is drawn perpendicular from the PCL to the posterior-most aspect of the H line.
- The *anorectal angle* is measured by drawing lines along the posterior border of the rectum and long axis of the anal canal.
- Pelvic organ prolapse can be graded by measuring the distance from the PCL (most common) or the midpubic line (MPL). The MPL approximates the level of the vaginal hymen, and is drawn along the long axis of the pubic symphysis.
- Cystocele is graded by the distance from the PCL/MPL to inferior bladder base (▶ Table 23.2 and ▶ Fig. 23.2).
- Uterine/vaginal prolapse is graded by the distance from the PCL/MPL to the anterior cervical lip or superior vaginal cuff, respectively (▶ Table 23.2).
- Cul-de-sac hernias include peritoneoceles, enteroceles, and sigmoidoceles, and are usually difficult to accurately diagnose clinically.
- *Anterior rectocele* is measured from the actual location of the anterior rectal wall to its expected location (approximated by the location of the anterior anal canal) at maximal strain (▶ Fig. 23.3). A bulge of < 2 cm is mild (and often asymptomatic), 2 to 4 cm is moderate, and > 4 cm is large.

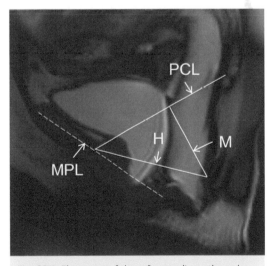

Fig. 23.1 Placement of the reference lines: the pubococcygeal line (PCL), midpubic line (MPL), H line (H), M line (M).

Table 23.1 Grading of pelvic floor relaxation using H and M lines

Grade	H Line (Hiatal widening)	M Line (Pelvic floor descent)
Normal	< 6 cm	< 2 cm
Mild	6–8 cm	2–4 cm
Moderate	8–10 cm	4–6 cm
Severe	> 10 cm	> 6 cm

Source: Adapted from Kobi et al 2018.[5]

Table 23.2 Grading of the pelvic organ prolapse

Reference: Pubococcygeal line		Reference: Midpubic line	
Distance from the organ to the PCL	Grade	Distance from the organ to the MPL	Stage
<1 cm below	Normal	>3 cm above	0
1–3 cm below	Mild	1–3 cm above	1
3–6 cm below	Moderate	Within 1 cm of the MPL (above or below)	2
>6 cm below	Severe	>1 cm below	3
		Complete organ eversion	4

Source: Adapted from Kobi et al 2018.[5]
Note: The distance is measured from the inferior bladder (cystocele), anterior inferior cervical lip (uterine prolapse), and superior vaginal cuff (vaginal prolapse).

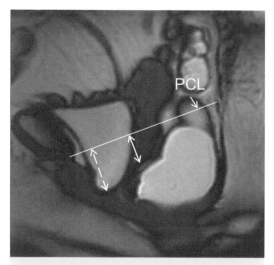

Fig. 23.2 Measurements of a cystocele (*dashed line*) and uterine prolapse (*solid line*). PCL, pubococcygeal line.

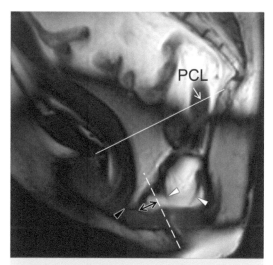

Fig. 23.3 Measurement of an anterior rectocele (*white line*). *Dashed white line* is the expected location of the anterior rectal wall (in line with the anterior anal canal). Note a large peritoneocele (*black arrowhead*) and mucosal intrarectal intussusception (*white arrowheads*).

- *Rectal intussusception* can be intrarectal (i.e., confined to the rectum), intra-anal (i.e., extend to the anal canal), or extra-anal (i.e., pass beyond the anal orifice). Intussusceptions can be mucosal (i.e., involving rectal mucosa only), or full-thickness (i.e., involve the entire wall).
- *Pelvic floor dyssynergia* results from failure of relaxation or paradoxical contraction of the

puborectalis during defecation. The findings include paradoxical decrease of the anorectal angle with defecation/maximal strain, and hypertrophy of the puborectalis.

References

[1] Flusberg M, Sahni VA, Erturk SM, Mortele KJ. Dynamic MR defecography: assessment of the usefulness of the defecation phase. AJR Am J Roentgenol. 2011; 196(4):W394–W399

[2] Attenberger UI, Morelli JN, Budjan J, et al. The value of dynamic magnetic resonance imaging in interdisciplinary treatment of pelvic floor dysfunction. Abdom Imaging. 2015; 40(7):2242–2247

[3] Broekhuis SR, Fütterer JJ, Barentsz JO, Vierhout ME, Kluivers KB. A systematic review of clinical studies on dynamic magnetic resonance imaging of pelvic organ prolapse: the use of reference lines and anatomical landmarks. Int Urogynecol J Pelvic Floor Dysfunct. 2009; 20(6):721–729

[4] García del Salto L, de Miguel Criado J, Aguilera del Hoyo LF, et al. MR imaging-based assessment of the female pelvic floor. Radiographics. 2014; 34(5):1417–1439

[5] Kobi M, Flusberg M, Paroder V, Chernyak V. Practical guide to dynamic pelvic floor MRI. J Magn Reson Imaging. 2018; 47 (5):1155–1170

24 Endometriosis MRI

Nicole Hindman

24.1 Template

Clinical indication: Endometriosis
Technique:
Using a torso phased-array coil, multiplanar T2-weighted images, axial diffusion-weighted images, axial 2D in-and-opposed-phase gradient-echo T1-weighted images, and pre- and postcontrast 3D sagittal and axial fat-suppressed gradient-echo T1-weighted images were obtained on a [1.5 T/3T] magnet. Vaginal gel was self-administered by the patient on the table. The patient was slowly injected with 0.9 mg of glucagon intravenously prior to acquisition of the T2-weighted images in order to minimize bowel peristalsis
Contrast: [___] mL of Gadavist
Comparison: [ ]
Findings:

- Uterus size: [____] [CC] × [____] [AP] × [____] [transverse] cm, volume [____] mL
- Junctional zone thickness: [ ] mm [normal/consistent with diffuse/focal adenomyosis]
- Adenomyomas: [no/yes, in the [posterior/anterior/fundal/corneal aspect of the uterus, measuring [__] cm]
- Fibroids: [no/yes, measuring [__] cm in [submucosal/intramural/subserosal] location, with [homogenous enhancement/heterogenous enhancement/no enhancement]]
- Cervix: [normal]
- Endometrium: [__] mm

Ovaries:
Right ovary: [CC] × [AP] × [transverse] cm for an overall volume of [__] mL. [Describe ovarian endometrioma/other findings.]
Left ovary: [CC] × [AP] × [transverse] cm for an overall volume of [__] mL
[Describe ovarian endometrioma/other findings]
Regions of thickening in the pelvis are described below:

Anterior compartment:

- Bladder: [normal/location and region of involvement (closeness to trigone)/tethering involving ____]
- Ureter: [normal/length of involvement (distance from bladder)/tethering involving____/describe hydroureter]
- Vesicouterine pouch: [normal/focal thickening/tethering involving____]
- Vesicovaginal pouch: [normal/focal thickening/tethering involving____]

Middle compartment:

- Uterine body: [normal/focal thickening/tethering involving____/mention cervical involvement]
- Fallopian tube: [normal/distended with high T2 signal content, likely fluid/with high T1 signal content, likely blood products]
- Uterine ligaments: [normal/thickened [right/left/both]

Posterior compartment:

- Uterosacral ligaments: [normal/thickened, [right/left/both]
- Rectovaginal septum: [normal/thickened, with/without rectal tethering]
- Anterior rectal wall: [normal/tethering with/without luminal invasion]
- Sigmoid colon: [normal/tethering to the uterus, with/without luminal invasion]
- Any other foci of involvement: [none/small bowel tethering/appendiceal involvement]
- Lymph nodes: [none/present—describe]
- Osseous structures: [no aggressive osseous lesion/present—describe]
- Additional findings: [none/describe]

Impression:
Imaging findings suspicious for deep endometriosis, with suspected [anterior/middle/posterior/tricompartmental] involvement

24.2 Stakeholders

Gynecologic surgeons, endometriosis specialist surgeons, general surgeons (colorectal), fertility specialists, and pain specialists.

24.3 Pearls

- A structured report tailored for known or suspected endometriosis can provide important information for treatment planning for multidisciplinary members of a treatment team, particularly for gynecologic and fertility physicians.[1,2]
- Endometriosis is a common gynecologic condition (estimated 10% prevalence in women of reproductive age), defined as the presence of endometrial glands and stroma outside the uterus.[3]
- There are no pathognomonic symptoms or biomarkers that are diagnostic of endometriosis. Most patients that are sent for imaging present with chronic pelvic pain or infertility.[4]
- Based on location and depth, endometriosis within the pelvis is classified intraoperatively as follows:
  - A superficial peritoneal lesion.
  - An ovarian endometrioma.
  - Deep endometriosis (endometriotic lesions extending more than 5 mm below the peritoneum).
- Superficial peritoneal lesions are occult on imaging; however, ovarian endometriomas and deep endometriosis can be detected on imaging, and knowledge of the extent of involvement is useful in determining appropriate therapy.[5]
- An ovarian endometrioma typically has uniformly high T1-W signal, with uniform loss of signal ("shading") on T2-W images. Another sign

of ovarian endometrioma is "*T2 dark spot*," which is a dependent focus of low signal on T2-W images, with a corresponding hyperintensity on T1-W images.
- The MR imaging features of deep endometriosis depends on the type of lesion: infiltrating small implants versus solid deep lesions. *Small infiltrating lesions* are typically low/intermediate signal on T1-W images and low signal on T2-W images, whereas *deep solid lesions* have low/intermediate signal intensity on T1-weighted images with or without foci of high signal, with corresponding diffuse low-signal intensity on T2-weighted images.
- Unless specifically trained, many general radiologists do not notice regions of deep endometriosis on pelvic MRI, and the structured report assists in the recognition of this common entity. Once recognized, this allows the clinicians to appropriately consider care options/ fertility options.
- Describing disease by compartment (anterior, middle, and posterior) helps the operative surgeon know the degree of dissection required (▶ Fig. 24.1).
- A thorough structured report is essential in showing all the potential sites of endometriotic disease, providing a road map for the operative surgeon, and for preoperative planning (for example, determining whether urology/ colorectal general surgery will need to be involved, for extensive bladder and bowel involvement, respectively) (▶ Fig. 24.2).
- The degree of disease suspected at MRI usually appears less severe than what is encountered intraoperatively. For example, ▶ Fig. 24.3 shows an MRI that demonstrates endometriosis in the anterior, middle, and posterior compartments. For the operative surgeon, this translates into a

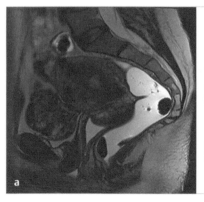 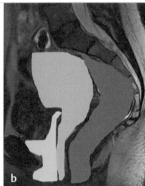

Fig. 24.1 Three-compartment model of deep endometriosis. **(a)** Sagittal T2-weighted image through the pelvis, after administration of vaginal gel and rectal gel. **(b)** The same image is shown, with the three compartments outlined in different shades: the anterior compartment is outlined in *white*, the middle compartment is *light gray*, and the posterior compartment is *dark gray*.

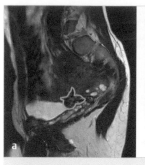
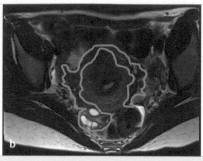
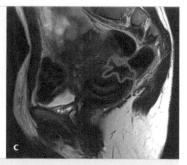

Fig. 24.2 Thirty-six-year-old woman with chronic pelvic pain, with tri-compartmental involvement by deep endometriosis. **(a)** Sagittal T2-weighted fast spin echo (FSE) image through the pelvis demonstrates low-signal intensity T2-weighted tethering in the anterior compartment (outlined). **(b)** Axial T2 FSE-weighted images through the pelvis demonstrate T2 plaques along the uterine body, tethering the ovaries to the uterus (regions of deep endometriosis in the middle compartment outlined). **(c)** Sagittal T2-weighted FSE images demonstrate thickening along the uterosacral ligaments (not shown) with thickening and fibrosis along the rectovaginal septum (outlined).

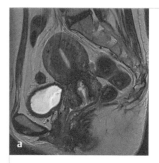
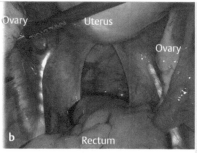
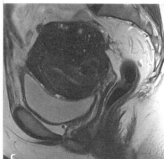
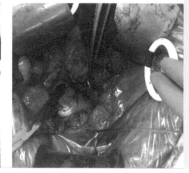

Fig. 24.3 Two different patients with corresponding intraoperative findings. Top row, 40F with history of pain, with sagittal T2 fast spin echo (FSE) **(a)** images showing a thickened junctional zone without evidence for deep endometriosis. Corresponding intraoperative laparoscopic image **(b)** demonstrating a normal appearance of the uterus, uterosacral ligaments, and ovaries. Bottom row, 37F with chronic pain, with sagittal T2 FSE **(c)** image showing diffuse adenomyosis of the uterus, as well as adhesions and thickening along the superior uterine body with tethering of the sigmoid colon (not shown) to the uterine body. Corresponding intraoperative open image **(d)** shows extensive bowel displaced into the pelvis, with multiple adhesions and lack of the normal fat planes of the pelvis, termed a "frozen pelvis" by surgeons.

completely "frozen" pelvis, a pelvis where all three compartments appear socked together without any visible fat plane between the compartments.

References

[1] Mattos LA, et al. Structured US and MRI imaging report for patients with suspected endometriosis: guide for imagers and clinicians. J Minim Invasive Gynecol. 2019; 26(6): 1016–1025

[2] Montoliu-Fornas G, Martí-Bonmatí L. Magnetic resonance imaging structured reporting in infertility. Fertil Steril. 2016; 105(6):1421–1431

[3] Bazot M, Bharwani N, Huchon C, et al. European Society of Urogenital Radiology (ESUR) guidelines: MR imaging of pelvic endometriosis. Eur Radiol. 2017; 27(7):2765–2775

[4] Agarwal SK, Chapron C, Giudice LC, et al. Clinical diagnosis of endometriosis: a call to action. Am J Obstet Gynecol. 2019; 220(4):354.e1–354.e12

[5] Coutinho A, Jr, Bittencourt LK, Pires CE, et al. MR imaging in deep pelvic endometriosis: a pictorial essay. Radiographics. 2011; 31(2):549–567

25 Cystic Pancreatic Lesions: Template for CT and MRI

Khoschy Schawkat and Koenraad J. Mortele

25.1 Template

Number of lesions: [single/multiple]
If [multiple]:
- The largest/dominant lesion should be measured if no worrisome imaging features are present
- Most worrisome imaging features of all lesions should be listed

Location: [uncinate process/head/neck/body/tail/outside]
Size (outer wall to outer wall): [longest dimension_ cm], which [plane][series][image number]
Prior measurement: [_ cm] [date of prior study]
Morphology: [round, oval, lobulated, elongated, pleomorphic, other], [multiloculated, uniloculated], [macrocystic, microcystic]
Wall: [thin, imperceptible/thick (> 3 mm)/perceptible]
(Pseudo)-Septations: [absent/present]
Solid mural nodule (> 3 mm): [absent/present]
If [present]: size [_ mm], enhancement [nonenhancing/likely enhancing/enhancing]
Calcification: [absent/present]
If [present]: [central/peripheral]
Communication with main pancreatic duct (MPD): [yes/no] [indeterminate]
MPD: [Nondilated] [Dilated: _ mm]
If [Dilated]: location [head/neck/body/tail/diffuse]
Mural nodule within MPD: [absent/present]
MPD wall thickening or enhancement: [absent/present]
Focal narrowing of pancreatic duct with parenchymal atrophy: [absent/present]
Remainder of pancreatic parenchyma: [unremarkable/describe abnormality]
Peripancreatic soft tissues: [unremarkable/edema/stranding/collection/other]
Biliary dilation: [absent/present]
Soft tissue mass in pancreas outside cyst: [location]

25.2 Stakeholders

Radiologists, gastroenterologists, oncologists, pathologists, and pancreaticobiliary surgeons.

25.3 Pearls

- Incidental pancreatic cystic lesions are categorized as benign lesions (e.g., pseudocysts or serous cystic tumors), or potentially malignant lesions (e.g., intraductal papillary mucinous neoplasms [IPMN] or mucinous cystic tumors).[1]
- Additional work-up of incidental pancreatic cysts is best performed with magnetic resonance imaging ± cholangiopancreatography (MRI/MRCP), if not applicable or available, with computed tomography (CT), or endoscopic ultrasound (EUS) with or without intervention.
- MRI is the preferred method for the investigation and follow-up of pancreatic cystic lesions.[2] 1.5 T or a 3 T MRI acquisition should be performed using phased-array coils to evaluate pancreatic cysts.
- Because the incidence of synchronous and metachronous pancreatic cancer is presumed higher in patients with pancreatic cysts, contrast-enhanced imaging is recommended to assess the entire pancreas in these patients.
- In patients with contraindications to MRI, multidetector CT (MDCT) with pancreatic protocol is an alternative. The advantage of MDCT over MRI is the easier availability, the possibility of image postprocessing in any planar reformation, and high spatial resolution (▶ Fig. 25.1).
- The MDCT pancreatic protocol should include a split-bolus protocol[3] or at least a dual-phase

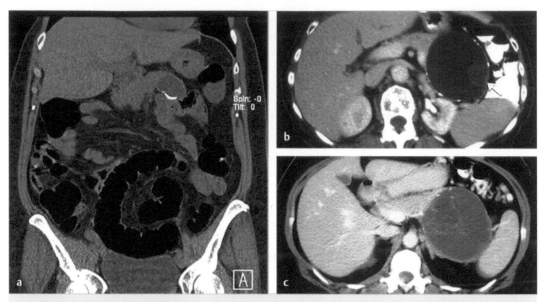

Fig. 25.1 Multidetector computed tomography in coronal plane without contrast **(a)** and in axial plane after intravenous contrast administration **(b and c)** demonstrating cystic pancreatic tail lesions with peripheral coarse calcification in **(a)** and focal wall calcifications in **(b)** and **(c)**. In **(b)** the cystic lesion shows a nonenhancing mural nodule (*arrow*) while in **(c)** multiple thin septations are demonstrated with one punctate septal calcification and several peripheral calcifications along the cystic wall in **(c)**. The main pancreatic duct is not dilated and the surrounding peripancreatic soft tissue is unremarkable. The findings are consistent with mucinous cystic neoplasms.

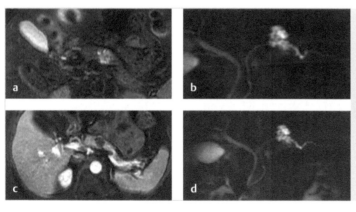

Fig. 25.2 T2-weighted fat saturated magnetic resonance (MR) image in axial orientation **(a)** shows a focal multiloculated cystic lesion in the pancreatic body/tail with upstream pancreatic main duct dilatation, best depicted on magnetic resonance cholangiopancreaticography (MRCP) **(b and d)**. After IV contrast administration **(c)** there is no evidence of an enhancing solid component. The findings are consistent with a serous microcystic adenoma.

contrast-enhanced acquisition in pancreatic and portal venous phases.

- Lesions should be measured in the longest dimension without measuring the narrow connection to main pancreatic duct (MPD).
- The true size/shape of these lesions is assessed through bidimensional measurement of the cysts. But the current guidelines for IPMN management and follow-up are based on the longest diameter only.
- If the cyst size is stable compared to the immediate prior study, but bigger compared to a remote study, include measurement and date from that particular remote study. Any intervention between the present and prior studies (e.g., aspiration) should be noted.
- At the level of the pancreatic head, an isolated finding of MPD caliber of 5 mm may be a normal variant (if there is no associated additional finding such as cystic lesion, abrupt duct caliber change, or interval change from prior imaging). However, the MPD upstream (in the pancreatic body and tail) should remain < 3 mm in diameter[4] (► Fig. 25.2).

- In IPMN, the revised international consensus Fukuoka guidelines consider the rate of cyst growth as worrisome if it is greater than 5 mm in 2 years[5] (▶ Table 25.1 and ▶ Table 25.2).
- The location of the lesion is important to report in order to allow localization during intervention and surgical planning, e.g., via EUS and to narrow the differential diagnosis.
- Assessment of the peripancreatic soft tissue is important as it may direct the differential diagnosis (signs of infiltrative neoplasm or signs of acute/chronic pancreatitis).

Table 25.1 Worrisome features and high-risk stigmata as defined by the revised Fukuoka guidelines in 2017[5]

Worrisome features	High-risk stigmata
Cyst size ≥ 3 cm Enhancing mural nodule < 5 mm Thickened enhancing cyst wall Abrupt change in the main pancreatic duct caliber with distal pancreatic atrophy Main pancreatic duct caliber 5–9 mm Rapid growth of the cyst > 5 mm/2 y Lymphadenopathy Elevated serum level of carbohydrate antigen (CA) 19-9	Enhancing solid component within cyst Main pancreatic duct caliber ≥ 10 mm in absence of obstruction Obstructed jaundice with cystic lesion in the pancreatic head

Table 25.2 Follow-up of IPMN cysts with no worrisome features or high-risk stigmata

Fukuoka guidelines	
< 1 cm	CT/MRI in 6 mo, then every 2 y if no change
1–2 cm	CT/MRI 6 mo × 1 y; yearly × for 2 y, then lengthen interval up to 2 y
2–3 cm	EUS in 3–6 mo, then lengthen interval up to 1 y, alternating MRI with EUS as appropriate. Consider surgery in young, fit patients
> 3 cm	Close surveillance alternating MRI with EUS every 3–6 mo. Strongly consider surgery in young, fit patients
ACR guidelines	
< 1.5 cm	• < 65 y at presentation: reimage yearly for 5 y and every 2 y for 4 y. Stop if stable for 9 y • 65–79 y at presentation: reimage every 2 y for 10 y. Stop if stable • > 80 y: reimage every 2 y for 4 y. Stop if stable
1.5–2.0 cm	• With established communication with MPD: reimage yearly for 5 y and every 2 y for 4 y. Stop if stable for 9 y or if cyst < 2.5 cm over 10 y • Communication with MPD cannot be established: Similar to management of 2.0–2.5 cm cyst • > 80 y: reimage every 2 y for 4 y. Stop if stable
2.0–2.5 cm	• Reimage every 6 mo for 2 y, then every year for 2 y and every 2 y for 6 y. Stop if stable for 10 y • > 80 y: reimage every 2 y for 4 y. Stop if stable
> 2.5 cm	• Low risk by imaging: similar to management of 2.0–2.5 cm cyst • High risk by imaging: EUS/FNA and surgical consultation • > 80 y: reimage every 2 y for 4 y. Stop if stable
AGA guidelines	
Cyst of any size with less than 2 positive features	Repeat MRI in 1 y and then every 2 y for 4 y. Stop surveillance if no positive features develop in 5 y

Abbreviations: ACR, American College of Radiology; AGA, American Gastroenterological Association; CT, computed tomography; EUS, endoscopic ultrasound; FNA, fine needle aspiration; IPMN, intraductal papillary mucinous neoplasms; MPD, main pancreatic duct; MRI, magnetic resonance imaging.

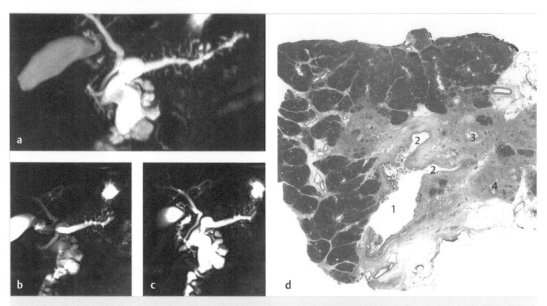

Fig. 25.3 (a–d) Magnetic resonance (MR) cholangiopancreaticography shows dilatation of the main pancreatic duct along the entire course with caliber irregularities in the pancreatic tail. Notably dilated side branches of the pancreatic duct in the pancreatic body and tail are seen. Histopathology reveals an intraductal papillary mucinous neoplasm involving the main duct (1), branch ducts (2), interlobular ducts (3), and intralobular ducts (4) with peritumoral chronic pancreatitis.

- In 2018, the European Study Group on Cystic Tumors of the Pancreas published evidence-based guidelines on pancreatic cystic neoplasms.[2] Their absolute indications for resection are positive cytology for malignancy, solid mass, presence of mural nodules (≥ 5 mm) and MPD dilatation of > 10 mm. The relative indications for resection are rapid increase in size (> 5 mm/y), new onset of diabetes mellitus, cystic diameter ≥ 40 mm and elevated serum CA 19–9 levels (▶ Fig. 25.3).

References

[1] Sahani DV, Kambadakone A, Macari M, Takahashi N, Chari S, Fernandez-del Castillo C. Diagnosis and management of cystic pancreatic lesions. AJR Am J Roentgenol. 2013; 200 (2):343–354

[2] Del Chiaro M, et al. European Study Group on Cystic Tumours of the Pancreas. European evidence-based guidelines on pancreatic cystic neoplasms. Gut. 2018; 67(5):789–804

[3] Brook OR, Gourtsoyianni S, Brook A, Siewert B, Kent T, Raptopoulos V. Split-bolus spectral multidetector CT of the pancreas: assessment of radiation dose and tumor conspicuity. Radiology. 2013; 269(1):139–148

[4] Mortelé KJ, Rocha TC, Streeter JL, Taylor AJ. Multimodality imaging of pancreatic and biliary congenital anomalies. Radiographics. 2007

[5] Tanaka M, Fernández-Del Castillo C, Kamisawa T, et al. Revisions of international consensus Fukuoka guidelines for the management of IPMN of the pancreas. Pancreatology. 2017; 17(5):738–753

26 Acute and Chronic Pancreatitis

Temel Tirkes

26.1 Template

Acute Pancreatitis

Pancreas:
- Necrosis: [none/head/body/tail] (Select all that apply)
- Percent of pancreatic necrosis: [none/< 30%/30–50%/> 50%]
- Peripancreatic collections: [acute peripancreatic fluid collection/pseudocyst/acute necrotic collection/ walled off necrosis] measuring [_] × [_] cm, extending to [__] compartment [with/without] gas within

Ductal system and gallbladder:
- Pancreatic duct caliber (largest): [ ] mm
- Biliary ductal diameter (largest): [ ] mm
- Choledocholithiasis: [absent/present]
- Gallbladder: [absent/normal wall thickness/thickened wall and with/without stones]

Vasculature:
- Venous thrombosis of splenic vein/SMV/portal vein: [absent/present]
- Portal/Splenic varices: [absent/present]
- Pseudoaneurysm: [absent/present in [_] vessel with/without evidence of active extravasation

Bowel:
- Bowel wall thickening: [absent/present]

Chronic Pancreatitis

Pancreas:
- Pancreatic parenchymal diameter: [ ] mm
- Pancreas involvement with abnormalities: [none/≤ 30%/30–70%/≥ 70%]
- Pancreas-to-splenic MR signal intensity ratio on precontrast T1-weighted image with fat suppression: [normal, > 1.2/decreased, ≤ 1.2]

Ductal system:
- Main pancreatic duct caliber (largest): [ ] mm
- Number of ectatic side-branch ducts: [none/< 3/≥ 3]
- Common bile duct caliber: [ ] mm
- Pancreatic duct stricture: [none/head/body/tail] (select all that apply)
- Parenchymal calcification: [absent/present]
- Intraductal calculus: [none/head/body/tail] (select all that apply)
- Pancreatic ductal stricture: [none/head/body/tail] (select all that apply)
- (Secretin MRCP) Duodenal filling grade: grade [0/1/2/3/4]

Gallbladder:
- Choledocholithiasis: [absent/present]
- Gallbladder: [absent/normal wall thickness/thickened wall and with/without stones]

Vasculature:
- Venous thrombosis of splenic vein/SMV/portal vein: [absent/present]
- Portal/Splenic varices: [absent/present]
- Pseudoaneurysm: [absent/present in [ ] vessel with/without evidence of active extravasation

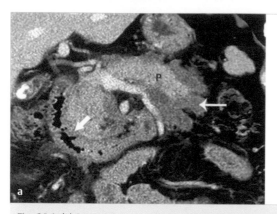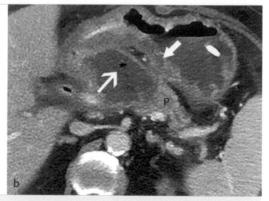

Fig. 26.1 **(a)** Pancreatitis in a 57-year-old woman. Coronal computed tomography (CT) obtained 5 weeks after acute episode shows a pseudocyst with well-defined rim surrounding the body and tail of the pancreas (*thin white arrow*). Pancreas (P) is homogenously enhancing. Duodenal folds are slightly thickened (*thick white arrow*). **(b)** Walled-off necrosis (WON) of pancreatic body and head. This is an axial contrast-enhanced CT image in a 45-year-old man with alcohol abuse. This CT was obtained 6 weeks after acute onset showed a heterogeneous collection replacing the parenchyma. The collection has a well-defined rim and gas bubble (*thin arrow*), representing a WON involving pancreas (P) and peripancreatic tissues. There is also thickening of gastric wall (*thick arrow*).

26.2 Stakeholders

Gastroenterologists, pancreatic surgeons, and interventional radiologists.

26.3 Pearls

- Contrast-enhanced computed tomography (CT) is best suited for staging in patients with acute pancreatitis, helping assess complications, and monitoring of treatment response through follow-up studies.[1,2]
- The revision of the Atlanta classification focuses heavily on morphologic criteria for defining the various manifestations of acute pancreatitis as outlined principally by means of CT.[1]
- Ductal morphology is better evaluated with magnetic resonance cholangiopancreatography (MRCP) than CT.[2,3]
- There are two types of acute pancreatitis: interstitial (edematous) and necrotizing pancreatitis, defined by revised Atlanta classification.[1]
- In patients with acute interstitial pancreatitis, CT and magnetic resonance imaging (MRI) demonstrates a localized or diffuse enlargement of the pancreas, with homogeneous enhancement or slightly heterogeneous enhancement of the pancreatic parenchyma.[1]
- Fluid collections are defined by timing from the onset of pancreatitis and presence of necrosis:

  - Acute peripancreatic fluid collections (in the first 4 weeks without necrosis).
  - Pseudocysts (encapsulated fluid collections after 4 weeks, without necrosis).
  - Acute necrotic collections (ANCs; in first 4 weeks, with necrosis).
  - Walled-off necrosis (WON; encapsulated collections after 4 weeks, with necrosis).[4]
- Intraparenchymal fluid collections due to pancreatitis are referred to as ANCs or WONs, not as pseudocysts (► Fig. 26.1).[4]
- Pseudocysts rarely become infected or require intervention; for sterile ANC or WON, any need for drainage is based on the clinical information; infected ANCs or WONs usually require intervention.[4]
- The ideal time for assessing acute pancreatitis complications with CT is after 72 hours from onset of symptoms. CT should be repeated when the clinical picture drastically changes, such as with sudden onset of fever, decrease in hematocrit, or sepsis.[4]
- Reporting standards of chronic pancreatitis that incorporates parenchymal and ductal abnormalities have been recently published.[5]
- Atrophy of the pancreas assessed by measuring thickness of pancreatic body at the left margin of the vertebral body and subtracting the ductal diameter if dilated.
- Parenchymal T1 signal intensity changes and parenchymal enhancement pattern during the

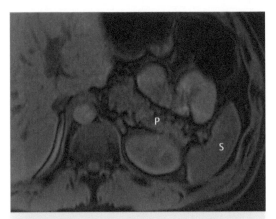

Fig. 26.2 Decreased T1-weighted signal of the pancreas. This is an axial precontrast, fat-suppressed T1-weighted gradient echo image in a 54-year-old female patient with suspected chronic pancreatitis. Normal T1-weighted signal of the pancreas (P) is greater than the spleen (S). In this patient with chronic pancreatitis, the signal intensity of the pancreas is less or same as the spleen.

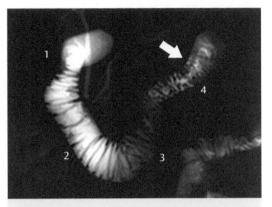

Fig. 26.3 Normal pancreatic juice excretion by secretin-enhanced magnetic resonance cholangiopancreatography (MRCP). This is a 10-minute postsecretin coronal MRCP image in a 39-year-old female being evaluated for chronic pancreatitis. The excreted pancreatic juice is filling the fourth portion of the duodenum (*arrow*) (grade 4) indicating normal response. Duodenal filling is graded according to the duodenal segments (1 to 4).

arterial and venous phases are features that have been shown to reflect tissue inflammation/fibrosis.[5]

- There is a correlation of pancreas signal intensity on the precontrast T1-weighted fat-suppressed gradient echo images with pancreatic exocrine function measured by the endoscopic pancreatic function tests. Pancreas-to-spleen signal intensity ratio less than 1.2 yields sensitivity of 77% and specificity of 83% for detection of pancreatic exocrine dysfunction, i.e., early chronic pancreatitis (▶ Fig. 26.2).[5]
- The exocrine fluid reserve of the pancreas can be assessed with secretin-enhanced MRCP. Fluid filling beyond the second portion of the duodenum (grade 2 or higher) is considered normal pancreatic excretion (▶ Fig. 26.3).[2]

References

[1] Banks PA, Bollen TL, Dervenis C, et al. Acute Pancreatitis Classification Working Group. Classification of acute pancreatitis—2012: revision of the Atlanta classification and definitions by international consensus. Gut. 2013; 62(1):102–111

[2] Conwell DL, Lee LS, Yadav D, et al. American Pancreatic Association Practice Guidelines in chronic pancreatitis: evidence-based report on diagnostic guidelines. Pancreas. 2014; 43(8):1143–1162

[3] Tirkes T, Sandrasegaran K, Sanyal R, et al. Secretin-enhanced MR cholangiopancreatography: spectrum of findings. Radiographics. 2013; 33(7):1889–1906

[4] Thoeni RF. The revised Atlanta classification of acute pancreatitis: its importance for the radiologist and its effect on treatment. Radiology. 2012; 262(3):751–764

[5] Tirkes T, Shah ZK, Takahashi N, et al. Consortium for the Study of Chronic Pancreatitis, Diabetes, and Pancreatic Cancer. Reporting standards for chronic pancreatitis by using CT, MRI, and MR cholangiopancreatography: the Consortium for the Study of Chronic Pancreatitis, Diabetes, and Pancreatic Cancer. Radiology. 2019; 290(1):207–215

27 Placenta Accreta Spectrum MRI

Priyanka Jha and Liina Poder

27.1 Template

Clinical history: EDD [ ] Cesarean section: [Numbers]. Other uterine instrumentation or relevant high-risk history: [ ]

Technique: Dedicated multiplanar T1- and T2-weighted, diffusion images were obtained through the placenta on a [1.5/3] T magnet

Findings:

Placental location: [ ]

Previa: [present/absent], [marginal/complete]

Placental findings:

- Heterogeneous placenta on T2 W images: [absent/present]
- T2 dark placental bands: [absent/[number]]
- Bulging of lower uterine segment: [absent/present]
- Loss of retroplacental clear space/myometrial thinning: [absent/present]
- Focal areas of myometrial invasion: [absent/anterior/posterior/lateral]
- Abnormal intraplacental and subplacental vascularity: [absent/present]
- Abnormal parametrial and bladder serosal vascularity: [absent/present]
- Urinary bladder invasion: [absent/present]
- Bulging of placenta into internal os: [absent/present]

Fetal position: [cephalic/breech/transverse]

Cervix: [closed/open]

Placental or amniotic hemorrhage on T1/diffusion imaging: [absent/present]

Other relevant observations: [ ]

Impression:

Level of suspicion for placenta accreta: [low/moderate/high]

Evidence for percreta and location, if present: [ ]

Other relevant observations: [ ]

27.2 Stakeholders

Obstetricians and gynecologists, gynecologic oncologists, interventional radiologist, urologists.

27.3 Pearls

- Placenta accreta spectrum (PAS) disorder includes a group of disorders characterized by abnormal placental attachment, and hence, the inability of the placenta to separate after delivery leading to catastrophic hemorrhage at the time of delivery. It is classified as *placenta accreta* (deep anchoring of the villi to decidua without myometrial invasion), *placenta increta* (with myometrial invasion present but intact uterine serosa) and *placenta percreta* (with full-thickness myometrial penetration beyond the serosa, with organ invasion to bladder and parametrium).[1]
- History of prior uterine instrumentation such as cesarean section delivery or dilation and curettage, which disrupts the endometrium, has been shown as the inciting risk factor. Additional risk factors include advanced maternal age, high gravity or parity, in vitro fertilization, prior uterine surgery and trauma, prior postpartum hemorrhage, Asherman syndrome, uterine anomalies (congenital or acquired), smoking, and hypertension.
- Magnetic resonance (MR) imaging has shown benefit over ultrasound in assessing the depth and topography of placental invasion, particularly for posterior placentas (▶ Fig. 27.1).[2]
- *Ideal gestational age to perform MRI* is between 28 and 32 weeks. After 32 weeks, myometrial

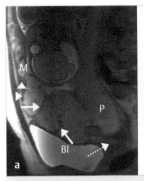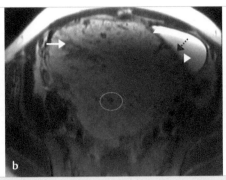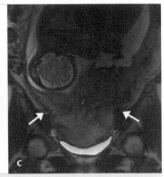

Fig. 27.1 Thirty-seven-year-old woman with history of five prior cesarean sections and placenta previa with increta and possibly percreta. **(a)** Sagittal T2-weighted non-fat-suppressed image of the uterus demonstrates complete placenta previa with the placenta (P) completely covering the internal os (*dotted arrow*). Multiple T2-dark bands are present, some of which are annotated by short arrows. **(b)** The placenta (P) abruptly bulges (*arrowheads*) into the myometrium (M) leading to placental bulge sign. Overlying myometrium is markedly thinned and almost imperceptible. **(b)** Axial T2-weighted non-fat-suppressed image demonstrates the marked heterogeneity of the placenta. Numerous T2-dark bands are present as well as abnormal intraplacental vascularity demonstrated by large branching flow voids (*circle*). Note the interface with the bladder, where the placenta is closely apposed to the bladder serosa, suspicious for 20 bladder invasion. There are flow voids present in the bladder wall (*arrowheads*), which are also predictive of bladder 21 invasion. **(c)** Coronal T2-weighted non-fat-suppressed image demonstrates all of these findings as well as an hourglass configuration to the uterus (*arrows*), another feature that is in keeping with placenta accreta spectrum disorder.

thinning from advancing gestation may lead to false-positive reads.

- Placental location should be recorded as anterior or posterior, along with an assessment for the presence of complete or marginal placenta previa. Presence of placenta previa or vasa previa precludes vaginal delivery and cesarean delivery becomes mandatory.
- PAS disorders usually present with a combination of imaging features and no single feature in isolation has been shown to be predictive of PAS disorders.[3,4,5]
- A combination of the following MR imaging features has been shown to occur in PAS disorders: T2-hypointense bands, heterogeneous placenta, placental bulge, placental ischemic infarction, asymmetric placental thickening, loss of retroplacental T2-hypointense line, myometrial thinning, abnormal intraplacental vascularity, abnormal placental bed vascularization, parametrial invasion, and/or bladder invasion.[2,3,4,5]
- Imaging-based distinction of placenta accreta, increta, and percreta has been challenging. Features such as placental bulge, serosal hypervascularity, abnormal vascularization of the placental bed, and parametrial hypervascularity are features suggestive of deeper invasive disease, including increta and percreta.[3,4]

- Bladder invasion and parametrial placental invasion are hallmark features of placenta percreta.[4,5]
- Intraplacental T2 dark bands, myometrial disruption, uterine bulge, and hypervascularity at the uteroplacental interface or parametrium portend poor clinical outcome for both mother and fetus.[5]
- Note should be made of unusual collaterals supplying the placental bed. While collaterals from the internal iliac artery are abundant, more severe cases may recruit collaterals from inferior epigastric arteries and other unusual locations. This information is important if interventional radiology-guided embolization is being considered to hemostasis.
- Abnormal vessels in the bladder dome, bladder tethering, and frank bladder invasion are suspicious for bladder invasion.[4,5] Preoperative cystoscopy may be contemplated and occasionally placement of ureteral stents will be required.
- Presence of deep invasive disease commits the patient to a cesarean hysterectomy in most cases in an attempt to control postpartum hemorrhage.[5] A number of fertility-sparing conservative management techniques has been reported, but not yet widespread in general practice.

References

[1] Familiari A, Liberati M, Lim P, et al. Diagnostic accuracy of magnetic resonance imaging in detecting the severity of abnormal invasive placenta: a systematic review and meta-analysis. Acta Obstet Gynecol Scand. 2018; 97(5):507–520

[2] Kilcoyne A, Shenoy-Bhangle AS, Roberts DJ, Sisodia RC, Gervais DA, Lee SI. MRI of placenta accreta, placenta increta, and placenta percreta: pearls and pitfalls. AJR Am J Roentgenol. 2017; 208(1):214–221

[3] Chen X, Shan R, Zhao L, et al. Invasive placenta previa: placental bulge with distorted uterine outline and uterine serosal hypervascularity at 1.5 T MRI—useful features for differentiating placenta percreta from placenta accreta. Eur Radiol. 2018; 28(2):708–717

[4] Bourgioti C, Zafeiropoulou K, Fotopoulos S, et al. MRI features predictive of invasive placenta with extrauterine spread in high-risk gravid patients: a prospective evaluation. AJR Am J Roentgenol. 2018; 211(3):701–711

[5] Bourgioti C, et al. MRI prognosticators for adverse maternal and neonatal clinical outcome in patients at high risk for placenta accreta spectrum (PAS) disorders. J Magn Reson Imaging. 2018

28 Ultrasound of Liver Transplant

S. Paran Yap and Ghaneh Fananapazir

28.1 Template

Donor type: [total liver, right lobe, left lobe, left lateral segment]
Grayscale:
Liver echogenicity: [normal/increased]
Liver echotexture: [normal/coarse]
Hepatic lesions: [none]
Perihepatic fluid collections: [none]
CBD diameter: [ ] mm

Color and spectral Doppler:
Hepatic artery
Flow is [present/absent]
Proximal (native) main hepatic artery:
- Peak systolic velocity: [ ] cm/s
- The resistive index: [ ]
- Parvus tardus waveform: [absent/present]

Arterial anastomosis:
- Peak systolic velocity: [ ] cm/s
- The resistive index: [ ]
- Parvus tardus waveform: [absent/present]

Distal (donor) main hepatic artery:
- Peak systolic velocity: [ ] cm/s
- The resistive index: [ ]
- Parvus tardus waveform: [absent/present]

Right hepatic artery:
- The resistive index: [ ]
- Parvus tardus waveform: [absent/present]

Left hepatic artery:
- The resistive index: [ ]
- Parvus tardus waveform: [absent/present]

Portal vein
Flow is [hepatopetal/hepatofugal/absent]
Peak systolic velocity:
- Proximal (native) main portal vein: [ ] cm/s
- Anastomosis: [ ] cm/s
- Distal (donor) portal vein: [ ] cm/s
- Right portal vein: [ ] cm/s with [hepatopetal/hepatofugal/absent] flow
- Left portal vein: [ ] cm/s with [hepatopetal/hepatofugal/absent] flow

Hepatic veins and IVC
Surgical anastomosis: [interposition/piggyback]
Spectral waveforms: [normal/abnormal]
Focal elevated velocity (> 3:1 ratio of elevated to unaffected venous velocity): [present/absent]

28.2 Stakeholders

Transplant surgeons, hepatologists, gastroenterologists, and interventional radiologists.

28.3 Pearls

- Liver grafts can come from deceased (most common) or living donors.
- Deceased grafts can either be transplanted as a whole or split into two separate grafts.
- There are four anastomotic sites: hepatic artery, caval, portal venous, and bile duct.
- Postoperative day 1 ultrasound is important for baseline measurements. Subsequent imaging is indicated for concerning clinical or laboratory findings.
- Ultrasound findings of acute rejection are nonspecific. Image-guided liver biopsy is important for the diagnosis of rejection.
- Surgically placed T-tube in the biliary system can mimic the appearance of thickened extrahepatic bile duct walls.
- A right-sided pleural effusion, mild ascites, perihepatic fluid, hematoma, and periportal edema can be normal postoperative findings.
- Hepatic artery waveform (▶ Fig. 28.1) should demonstrate brisk systolic upstroke and continuous diastolic flow. Time to peak systolic flow from start of upstroke (normal < 80 ms) and the resistive index (normal 0.5–0.7) should be obtained.
- Parvus tardus is seen distal to a hepatic artery stenosis and is defined as an acceleration time > 0.08 seconds.
- Portal venous waveforms should show continuous flow toward the liver.

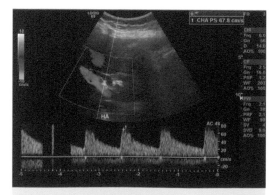

Fig. 28.1 Normal hepatic artery velocity and waveform.

- Caval vasculature should have a phasic waveform corresponding to the cardiac cycle.
- Hepatic artery thrombosis is a relatively common but devastating complication and will typically manifest as biliary dysfunction due to absent arterial perfusion, with later formation of biliary strictures and biliary necrosis. This is an urgent finding as it can be treated with endovascular or surgical approach to save the graft if detected early.
- Hepatic artery thrombosis is suggested by nonvisualization of hepatic artery on color and spectral Doppler. The resistive index (RI) of the main hepatic artery may be elevated proximal to the thrombosed segment. False-positive thromboses by ultrasound can occur owing to operator dependency (failed visualization), arterial spasms, and poor cardiac output. Contrast ultrasound, computed tomography (CT), and magnetic resonance (MR) angiography can be used to confirm ultrasound findings.
- Hepatic artery stenosis is suggested based on an elevated main hepatic artery peak systolic velocity (> 200 cm/s) and/or intrahepatic arteries with low-resistive indices and parvus tardus waveforms. Parvus tardus waveforms can also be found in long-term hepatic artery stenosis with collateral vessel formation, portal vein thrombosis, and atherosclerotic disease (▶ Fig. 28.2).
- Pseudoaneurysms of the hepatic artery occurs in up to 2% of transplants. These are round and anechoic structures with disorganized or bidirectional flow that may resemble a yin-yang symbol on color Doppler.
- Portal vein stenosis may result from donor/portal vessel mismatch and is diagnosed when peak anastomotic velocity exceeds 125 cm/s or is greater than a 3:1 anastomotic-to-preanastomotic velocity ratio (▶ Fig. 28.3).
- Inferior vena cava (IVC)/hepatic vein stenosis may occur at the anastomotic site or due to external compression. It is diagnosed when there is at least threefold increase in velocity and distension of hepatic veins proximal to site of stenosis. There will be a replacement of normal triphasic hepatic vein with monophasic waveforms. It is more common in living donor transplants.
- IVC/hepatic vein thrombosis can occur as a direct surgical complication or due to hypercoagulable state and will show an absence of flow.

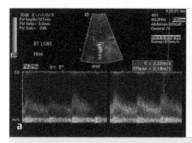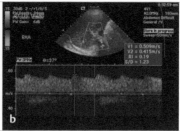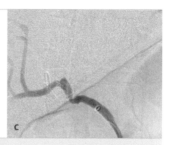

Fig. 28.2 **(a)** Transplant hepatic artery stenosis showing elevated arterial velocity. **(b)** Transplant hepatic artery stenosis showing low-resistive index and parvus tardus waveforms in the intrahepatic arteries, distal to the stenosis. **(c)** Transplant hepatic artery stenosis as shown on digital subtraction angiography.

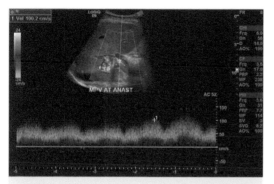

Fig. 28.3 Portal venous stenosis at the anastomosis demonstrating elevated velocity. The preanastomotic portal venous velocity was 30 cm/s.

- Biliary complications include strictures, leaks, bilomas, and stones and usually occur in the first 6 months.
- Patients with biliary stricture/stenosis may be clinically asymptomatic but demonstrate abnormal laboratory results. On ultrasound, the duct may be dilated; however, this feature is not sensitive, as 71% of patients with biliary strictures demonstrated nondilated bile ducts.
- Peritransplant collections include hematomas, bilomas, and abscesses.
- Malignancies in liver grafts include hepatocellular carcinoma, post-transplant lymphoproliferative disease, and angiosarcomas.

Suggested Readings

College of Radiology A. ACR–AIUM–SPR–SRU practice parameter for the performance of an ultrasound examination of solid organ transplants; ACR–AIUM–SPR–SRU practice parameter for the performance of an ultrasound examination of solid organ transplants. https://www.acr.org/-/media/ACR/Files/Practice-Parameters/SolidOrgan-Trans.pdf. Accessed February 14, 2019

Crossin JD, Muradali D, Wilson SR. US of liver transplants: normal and abnormal. Radiographics. 2003; 23(5):1093–1114

da Silva RF, Raphe R, Felício HC, et al. Prevalence, treatment, and outcomes of the hepatic artery stenosis after liver transplantation. Transplant Proc. 2008; 40(3):805–807

Novogrodsky E, Felker ER, Lu DSK, Raman SS. Imaging of liver transplantation. In: Transplantation imaging. Cham: Springer International Publishing; 2018:47–79

Singh AK, Nachiappan AC, Verma HA, et al. Postoperative imaging in liver transplantation: what radiologists should know. Radiographics. 2010; 30(2):339–351

29 Kidney Transplant

Kathryn McGillen and Ghaneh Fananapazir

29.1 Template

Comparison: [ ]
Transplant kidney:
The kidney is located in the [right lower quadrant/left lower quadrant]
Length: [ ] cm, previously [ ] cm
Echogenicity: [normal/increased/decreased]
Collecting system:
Hydronephrosis: [none/mild/moderate/severe], [stable/improved/worsened]
Urothelial thickening: [present/absent]
Bladder:
[Normal for degree of distention/limited evaluation due to underdistention/abnormal]
Perinephric space:
Fluid collection: [none/anechoic/homogeneous/heterogeneous/septations], measuring [ ] × [ ] × [ ] cm
[with/without] mass effect upon the kidney

Vascular Evaluation

Parenchymal perfusion: [normal/decreased/absent]
Native inflow artery: [internal/external] iliac artery with peak systolic velocity proximal to anastomosis
[ ] cm/s
Transplant renal artery: [not visualized/patent on color Doppler] with peak systolic velocity of
[ ] cm/sand [normal/absent diastolic flow/reversal of flow during diastole] waveform
Transplant renal vein: [not visualized/patent on color Doppler]
Intrarenal vasculature: Color Doppler—[normal/abnormal]
  - Intrarenal arteries (interlobar/segmental) resistive indices:
    - Upper pole [ ] – [ ] [low/normal/elevated]
    - Interpolar: [ ] – [ ] [low/normal/elevated]
    - Lower pole: [ ] – [ ] [low/normal/elevated]
  - Parvus tardus: [present/absent]

29.2 Stakeholders

Transplant surgeons, nephrologists, vascular surgeons, and interventional radiologists.

29.3 Pearls

- Perfusion should be demonstrated in the renal cortex (▶ Fig. 29.1). Decreased perfusion can be seen in the setting of acute tubular necrosis, rejection, renal vein thrombosis, and pyelonephritis.[1,2] Absent perfusion implies an arterial thrombosis.
- Mild dilation of the collecting system may be normal in kidney grafts owing to reflux and loss of ureteral tone from denervation. Comparison

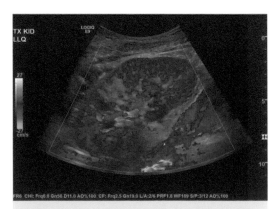

Fig. 29.1 Normal color Doppler perfusion of a left lower quadrant renal transplant.

for interval change is useful in determining if the dilation represents hydronephrosis.[2,3]

- Hydronephrosis can be caused by ureteral strictures or obstructing stones. Since the kidney is denervated, patients with hydronephrosis from obstructing stones may not experience pain and often present with elevated creatinine.[1,4]
- Urothelial thickening within the collecting system can be seen in the setting of infection, acute tubular necrosis, or rejection. The presence of debris may indicate hematuria or pyuria.[1,3]
- Hematomas are the most common peritransplant collection. Other collections include urinomas, seromas, abscesses, or lymphoceles. The etiology of the fluid collection can be suggested based on the post-transplant time course (► Table 29.1 and ► Fig. 29.2).[1,2,4]
- Small hematomas usually resolve on their own. However, larger hematomas often need to be evacuated due to (1) mass effect on the kidney or (2) their propensity to serve as a nidus for infection.[3]
- Transplant renal artery stenosis, the most common vascular complication (up to 10%), most often occurs within the first year post-transplant (► Fig. 29.3).[1,2,4]
- The normal velocity of the renal artery can be as high as 400 cm/s in the immediate postoperative setting. However, normal values usually range between 200 and 300 cm/s in the immediate postoperative period. Additional signs of

Table 29.1 Common perinephric collections and their sonographic characteristics

	Time after transplant	Characteristics	Treatment
Hematoma	Immediate postoperative	Heterogeneous Avascular Septations if chronic	Conservative unless large, mass effect upon kidney, or superinfection
Urinoma	< 2 wk	Anechoic No septations Well defined Rapidly increases	Percutaneous drainage Percutaneous nephrostomy with stent Surgical
Lymphocele	> 4–8 wk	Often medial to the transplant Anechoic +/– septations, thin wall	Most require no treatment Percutaneous aspiration if mass affect, causing obstruction, or superinfection Definitive treatment may require sclerotherapy
Abscess	At any time	Variable May be complex, cystic, thick walled, gas-containing	Antibiotics Percutaneous drainage Surgical—last resort

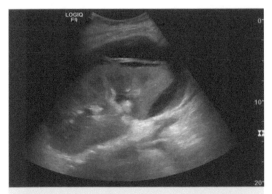

Fig. 29.2 Peritransplant collection—hematoma in the acute postoperative periods with mass effect upon the inferior pole. Acute hematomas can frequently be hyperechoic. This hematoma subsequently became superinfected.

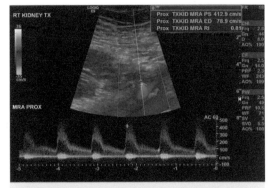

Fig. 29.3 Elevated peak systolic velocity in the main renal artery in a right lower quadrant renal transplant.

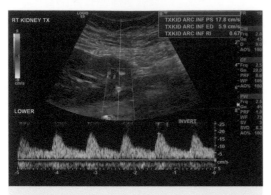

Fig. 29.4 Normal intrarenal (arcuate artery) resistive index in a right lower quadrant transplant kidney.

stenosis include turbulent flow distal to the stenosis and parvus tardus waveforms in the intraparenchymal arteries.[3,4]

- Interlobar arteries or segmental arteries are used in evaluating intrarenal vasculature resistive indices (RI) (▶ Fig. 29.4).
- Thresholds for RI are low < 0.6, normal 0.6–0.79, elevated > 0.79.
- *Low RIs* (< 0.6) can be seen in the setting of transplant renal artery stenosis and arteriovenous fistulas.
- *High RIs* (> 0.79) can be seen in the setting of rejection, acute tubular necrosis,

glomerulosclerosis, venous thrombosis, and graft compression by peritransplant collections.[5]

- *Renal vein thrombus* is uncommon (< 5%), but when present usually occurs within the first two postoperative weeks. Associated findings include enlarged, edematous kidney, reduced or absent venous flow in the vein, unidentifiable main renal vein, and reversed diastolic flow in the main renal artery.[1,4]
- Intrarenal arteriovenous fistula or pseudoaneurysms are often iatrogenic from biopsies. Treatment is often required only if large or symptomatic.[1,2]

References

[1] Brown ED, Chen MY, Wolfman NT, Ott DJ, Watson NE, Jr. Complications of renal transplantation: evaluation with US and radionuclide imaging. Radiographics. 2000; 20(3):607–622

[2] Kolofousi C, Stefanidis K, Cokkinos DD, Karakitsos D, Antypa E, Piperopoulos P. Ultrasonographic features of kidney transplants and their complications: an imaging review. ISRN Radiol. 2012; 2013:480862

[3] Galgano SJ, Lockhart ME, Fananapazir G, Sanyal R. Optimizing renal transplant Doppler ultrasound. Abdom Radiol (NY). 2018; 43(10):2564–2573

[4] Akbar SA, Jafri SZ, Amendola MA, Madrazo BL, Salem R, Bis KG. Complications of renal transplantation. Radiographics. 2005; 25(5):1335–1356

[5] Lockhart ME, Wells CG, Morgan DE, Fineberg NS, Robbin ML. Reversed diastolic flow in the renal transplant: perioperative implications versus transplants older than 1 month. AJR Am J Roentgenol. 2008; 190(3):650–655

30 Living Donor Liver Transplant

Jeffrey L. Weinstein, Robert Fisher, and Muneeb Ahmed

30.1 Template

Liver:
Liver border: [smooth/nodular]
Focal and diffuse liver disease:
Parenchyma: [normal/(mild, moderate, severe steatosis, [with/without] focal fat or fatty sparing)
Liver lesions: [none/(specify size, segment, and imaging characteristics)]
Liver volume: [total liver ____mL/donor lobe (right/left)____mL]
Arteries:
- **Celiac:** [no stenosis or aneurysm, median arcuate ligament compression]
- **Common hepatic artery:** [patent, arises from celiac/patent, arises from superior mesenteric artery]
- **Gastroduodenal artery:** [patent]
- **Proper hepatic artery:** [patent without stenosis or vascular abnormality]
- **Right hepatic artery:** [single, patent right hepatic artery from proper hepatic artery with normal branching/[accessory/replaced] right hepatic artery from the superior mesenteric artery]
- **Left hepatic artery:** [single, patent left hepatic artery from proper hepatic artery with normal branching/[accessory/replaced] left hepatic artery off of the left gastric artery]
- **Segment IV arterial supply:** [supply to segment IV arises off of the [right/left/right and left] hepatic artery] [the segment IV originates __cm from the origin of the right hepatic artery (for cases of segment IV supply off of the right hepatic artery)]

Veins:
- **Hepatic veins:** [Patent] [there are/are no accessory hepatic veins [if present, report diameter]]
- **Middle hepatic vein:** [distance from vena cava to first branch of middle hepatic vein ____.] [There are/are no branches from segment IV that drain into the middle hepatic vein.]
- **Right hepatic vein:** [type_____ ramification of the right hepatic vein]
- **Accessory right hepatic vein:** [no accessory right hepatic vein present/accessory right hepatic vein present, which is ____cm from the right hepatic vein in the coronal plane]
- **Portal vein:** [patent with normal branching/absence of the right portal vein/trifurcation of the portal vein/direct origin of the right anterior portal vein from left portal vein/absence of left portal vein/left portal arising from anterior branch of right portal vein]
- **Main portal vein diameter:** ___mm
- **Right portal vein diameter:** ___mm
- **Distance from the right portal vein to anterior/posterior bifurcation:** ___ mm
- **Origin of segment IV portal vein:** [from right/left portal vein, or both]
- **Biliary tree:** [conventional biliary anatomy/aberrant right posterior duct off of left/trifurcation of ducts/accessory ducts], [the biliary tree is free of calculi]

General:
- **Ascites:** [none/small/moderate/large]
- **Spleen size:** [normal/enlarged] [__cm in longest dimension]
- **Gallbladder:** [absent/present and [normal/distended/cholelithiasis noted]]

30.2 Stakeholders

Liver transplant surgeons, interventional radiologists, and transplant hepatologists.

30.3 Pearls

- Steatosis greater than 30% in a donor liver may result in dysfunction post-transplant in the graft.

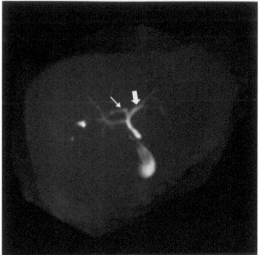

Fig. 30.1 Magnetic resonance cholangiopancreatography (MRCP) image depicting the right posterior duct (*thin arrow*) arising off of the left bile duct (*thick arrow*).

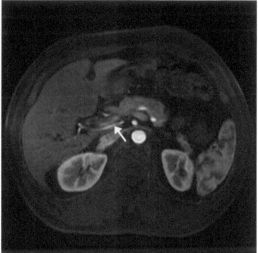

Fig. 30.2 Replaced right hepatic artery (*arrow*) off of the superior mesenteric artery coursing posterior to the portal vein.

- A liver remnant of 30 to 40% is needed post donation to ensure proper liver function. The remnant liver needs to be larger if there is underlying parenchymal liver disease such as steatosis.
- Approximately 40% of volume of the normal liver, as estimated by body surface area (BSA), is needed to maintain adequate function in the recipient:
  Liver volume (mL) = 706.2 × BSA (m²) + 2.4.
- *Standard biliary anatomy* is present in 58% of the population where anterior and posterior right ducts join to form a right duct and the segment IV and 2–3 ducts join to form a left duct.
- A right posterior biliary duct joining the left hepatic duct occurs in 13 to 19% of the population (▶ Fig. 30.1) and a trifurcation or triple confluence is seen in 11% of patients.
- Noting accessory and aberrant ducts is important for surgical planning. A transected bile duct can lead to a bile leak and an inadvertently ligated duct can lead to segmental atrophy.
- Livers with multiple arteries to the segment to be donated are typically avoided due to the surgical complexity of transplantation in these cases.
- When the hepatic artery arises off of the superior mesenteric artery (replaced/accessory right hepatic artery), the artery often runs deep to the portal vein and this may significantly alter the surgical approach (▶ Fig. 30.2).
- Segment IV of the liver is supplied by the right hepatic artery in approximately 11% of cases.
- The distance between a segment IV artery and the origin of the right hepatic artery is of clinical importance when segment IV is supplied by the right hepatic artery.
- A hepatic artery ≤ 3 mm may be too small to provide adequate arterial perfusion to the donor graft.
- Absence of the right portal vein occurs in 16.5% of patients and is often seen with a trifurcation of the portal vein.
- A portal vein trifurcation and a left portal vein arising from a branch of the right portal vein are relative contraindications to liver donation (▶ Fig. 30.3).
- Presence of large accessory hepatic veins (≥5 mm) (▶ Fig. 30.4) should be reported because they may need to be anastomosed individually to avoid venous congestion of the liver.
- An accessory inferior right hepatic vein, which is seen in 47 to 68% of patients, is of particular importance because if its distance from the true right hepatic vein is greater than 4 cm, it may present greater challenges with the surgical implantation.

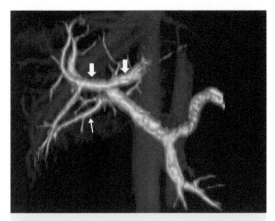

Fig. 30.3 Portal vein reconstruction where right anterior portal vein and left portal vein (*thick arrows*) arising separately from the right posterior portal vein (*thin arrow*). This type of anatomic variant has important surgical planning implications and should be described in the report.

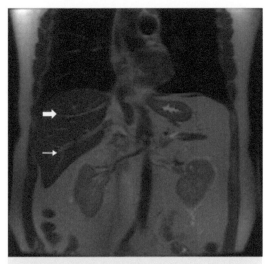

Fig. 30.4 Coronal T2 image showing the presence of an accessory right inferior hepatic vein (*thin arrow*) and right hepatic vein (*thick arrow*).

- The biliary anatomy can be classified by Huang et al as:
  A. Traditional classification of bile ducts with right anterior and posterior draining into right and then joining left.
  B. Trifurcation of bile ducts.
  C. Right posterior duct bent behind the right anterior duct as it joins the left duct.
  D. Separate, low branching of the right posterior segmental duct.
- Right hepatic venous ramification anatomy is classified as following:
  ○ Type 1 with no ramification (branching) in the first centimeter from the inferior vena cava.
  ○ Type 2a if the right superior vein branch comes off in the first centimeter.
    ○ Type 2b if the right anterosuperior vein comes off in the first centimeter.
  ○ Type 3 if both veins come off in the first centimeter.
  ○ Type 4 if there are separate ostia of the superior branch and main right hepatic vein.

Suggested Readings

Erbay N, Raptopoulos V, Pomfret EA, Kamel IR, Kruskal JB. Living donor liver transplantation in adults: vascular variants important in surgical planning for donors and recipients. AJR Am J Roentgenol. 2003; 181(1):109–114

Goyen M, Barkhausen J, Debatin JF, et al. Right-lobe living related liver transplantation: evaluation of a comprehensive magnetic resonance imaging protocol for assessing potential donors. Liver Transpl. 2002; 8(3):241–250

Hwang S, Lee SG, Sung KB, et al. Long-term incidence, risk factors, and management of biliary complications after adult living donor liver transplantation. Liver Transpl. 2006; 12(5):831–838

Mortelé KJ, Cantisani V, Troisi R, de Hemptinne B, Silverman SG. Preoperative liver donor evaluation: Imaging and pitfalls. Liver Transpl. 2003; 9(9):S6–S14

Urata K, Kawasaki S, Matsunami H, et al. Calculation of child and adult standard liver volume for liver transplantation. Hepatology. 1995; 21(5):1317–1321

Section IV

Structured Reports in Thoracic Imaging

Editors: Jonathan H. Chung and Diana Litmanovich

IV

31 Incidental Pulmonary Nodules

Milena Petranovic and Carol Wu

31.1 Template

Number of nodules: [single/multiple < 10 or/multiple > 10]
For each nodule (up to 5 most concerning nodules):
Attenuation: [solid/subsolid, pure ground-glass/subsolid, part-solid]
Presence of fat (−50 to −150 HU): [yes/no]
Presence of calcification (> 200 HU): [yes/no]
    If yes, pattern of calcification: [benign (diffuse, central, laminar, popcorn)/nonspecific (punctate, eccentric, amorphous)]
Presence of cavitation: [yes/no]
Size: [ ] (mean measurement of long and short axis; for part-solid nodules both the mean diameter of entire nodule as well as of solid component should be recorded)
Evolution: [stable/enlarging/decreasing/fluctuating]
Margins: [spiculated/smooth/irregular/ill-defined]
Shape: 2D: [round/oval/triangular/lobular, irregular] 3D: [spherical/flat]
Lobar location: [right upper lobe/right middle lobe/right lower lobe/left upper lobe/lingula/left lower lobe]
Perifissural: [yes/no]
Recommendation: [ ] (Based on the 2017 Fleischner Guidelines for the most suspicious nodule)

31.2 Stakeholders

Radiologists, thoracic surgeons, pulmonologists, and primary care physicians.

31.3 Pearls

- Pulmonary nodule is defined as a rounded or irregular opacity measuring up to 3 cm in diameter.
- Nodule evaluation is ideally performed on thin section computed tomography (CT) (slice thickness of 0.5–1.5 mm).
- *Nodule size* is expressed as the mean measurement of long- and short-axis measurements, obtained on the same axial, coronal, or sagittal image based on the largest size of nodule. For subsolid nodules, both the mean diameter of the entire nodule as well as the mean diameter of the solid component should be recorded (▶ Fig. 31.1).
- Approach to pulmonary nodule should include consideration of *nodule mimics*, multidisciplinary assessment, and further imaging/work-up as appropriate as well as adherence to 2017 Fleischner Guidelines for incidental nodules (▶ Fig. 31.2 and ▶ Table 31.1).
- Fleischner Society Guidelines do not apply to lung cancer screening, patients with immunosuppression, or patients with known primary cancer.
- There are many etiologies of lung nodules, both benign and malignant (▶ Table 31.2).
- To make a reliable diagnosis of hamartoma on CT, the density measurement of the lesion should be below negative 50 HU.
- Lung cancer tends to occur most frequently in the right upper lobe.
- Perifissural nodules are most frequently benign.
- *Spiculated contour or margin* has a positive predictive value for malignancy of 90%. While in general benign nodules tend to have a smooth contour, up to *20% of primary lung malignancies also have smooth margins.*
- Malignant solid pulmonary nodules usually have doubling time <100 days (typical range 20–400 d). Malignant subsolid nodule, however, may show a much more indolent growth pattern with doubling time up to several years. An increase in attenuation of a subsolid nodule is as concerning for malignancy as is an increase in size. Infectious/inflammatory causes often have a doubling time < 20 days.
- *Temporary decrease in size* has been reported in some cancers, possibly due to fibrosis or atelectasis or resolution of superimposed inflammatory component.

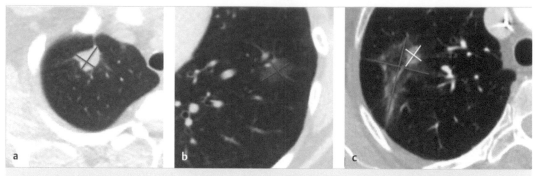

Fig. 31.1 **(a)** In the Fleischner guidelines, the nodule dimension using 2D caliper measurements should be based on the average of the long-axis and short-axis diameters and averaged to the nearest millimeter. **(b)** Like the solid nodule, a pure ground-glass nodule should also be measured as the average of the long-axis and short-axis diameters and averaged to the nearest millimeter. **(c)** For a part-solid nodule, both the total size of the nodule (gray calipers) as well as the size of the largest solid component (white calipers) should be measured separately. Both the total size and largest solid component should be measured as long and short axes and rounded to the nearest millimeter.

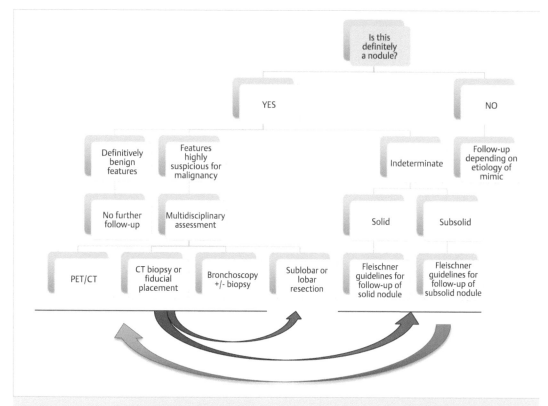

Fig. 31.2 General approach to the pulmonary nodule.

- Cystic nodules are not separately addressed in the Fleischner guidelines. Irregular nodular thickening of a cyst wall or interval development of a solid component is worrisome for malignancy within these nodules (▶ Fig. 31.3).

- Air-bronchogram can be seen in association with certain infections, pulmonary lymphoma, as well as in lung adenocarcinoma.
- Effort should be made to obtain and compare to oldest study available to detect slowly enlarging neoplasms.

Table 31.1 Guidelines for management of incidentally detected solid and subsolid pulmonary nodules in adults

Solid nodule follow-up guidelines		
	Size < 6 mm (< 100 mm³)	Size 6–8 mm (100–250 mm³)	Size > 8 mm (> 250 mm³)
Single nodule	No routine follow-up for low-risk patients[a] Optional CT at 12 months for high-risk patients[a]	CT at 6–12 mo (low- and high-risk patients) CT at 18–24 mo for high-risk patients (optional for low-risk patients)	CT, PET/CT, or tissue sampling at 3 mo (low- and high-risk patients)
Multiple nodules		CT at 3–6 mo (low- and high-risk patients) Another follow-up CT at 18–24 mo for high-risk patients (optional for low-risk patients)	

Subsolid nodule follow-up guidelines		
	Size < 6 mm (< 100 mm³)	Size ≥ 6 mm (≥ 100 mm³)
Single nodule	No routine follow-up[b]	Ground-glass: CT at 6–12 mo, then every 2 y until 5 y if persistent Part solid: CT at 3–6 mo, then annually until 5 y[c]
Multiple nodules	CT at 3–6 mo If stable, consider CT at 2 and 4 y	CT at 3–6 mo If persistent, subsequent management based on most suspicious nodule(s)

Source: Adapted from Fleischner Society 2017.
[a]Nodules < 6 mm do not require routine follow-up but certain patients at high-risk with suspicious nodule morphology, upper lobe location, or both may warrant 12-mo follow-up.
[b]In certain suspicious nodules < 6 mm, consider follow-up at 2 and 4 y and if solid component or growth develops, consider resection.
[c]Any persistent part-solid nodule with solid components ≥ 6 mm should be considered highly suspicious.

Table 31.2 Benign and malignant etiologies for solid and subsolid nodules

	Benign	Malignant
Solid nodule	Calcified and noncalcified granulomas	Lung cancer
	Scar	
	Intraparenchymal lymph node	Metastasis
	Hamartoma	Carcinoid
	Amyloidoma[b]	Lymphoma
	Rheumatoid nodule[b]	
	Organizing pneumonia	
Subsolid nodule	Infectious/inflammatory etiology[a] • Fungal pneumonia • Vasculitis • Aspiration	Adenocarcinoma spectrum Kaposi sarcoma[b]
	Organizing pneumonia	Lymphoproliferative disorder
	Focal interstitial fibrosis	
	Hemorrhage[a]	
	Endometriosis[b]	

[a]These are often transient subsolid nodules.
[b]Less common etiologies.

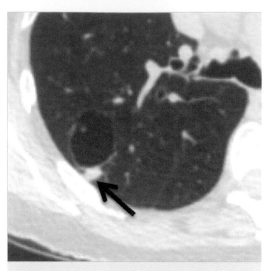

Fig. 31.3 Irregular or nodular thickening of a wall of a cyst (*arrow*) is worrisome for malignancy, in this case an adenocarcinoma.

Suggested Readings

ACR Data Science Institute use cases template. https://www.acrdsi.org/DSI-Services/TOUCH-AI

Bueno J, Landeras L, Chung JH. Updated Fleischner Society Guidelines for managing incidental pulmonary nodules: common questions and challenging scenarios. Radiographics. 2018; 38 (5):1337–1350

MacMahon H, Naidich DP, Goo JM, et al. Guidelines for management of incidental pulmonary nodules detected on CT images: from the Fleischner Society 2017. Radiology. 2017; 284(1):228–243

Petranovic M, Digumarthy SR. Incidental pulmonary nodule in thoracic imaging: the requisites (3rd ed.). Philadelphia: Elsevier Inc; 2019

32 CT Pulmonary Angiography

Brett W. Carter

32.1 Template

Technique:
The examination is [adequate/suboptimal/nondiagnostic] for the evaluation of the pulmonary arteries.
Pulmonary embolism:
There is [evidence/no evidence] of pulmonary embolism. A pulmonary embolus is present in the [right/left] [main/segmental/subsegmental] pulmonary artery.
Pulmonary arteries:
The pulmonary arteries are [normal in caliber/enlarged]. The pulmonary trunk, left main pulmonary artery, and right main pulmonary artery measure [ ] cm, [ ] cm, and [ ] cm, respectively.
Right heart strain:
There is [evidence/no evidence] of right heart strain. The right ventricle-to-left ventricle ratio is [ ], which [is/is not] suggestive of right heart strain.
Pulmonary Infarction:
There is [evidence/no evidence] of pulmonary infarction.
Lungs and airways:
The lungs are otherwise clear. The central airways are patent.
Pleura:
There is no evidence of pleural effusion or pneumothorax.
Heart and mediastinum:
The heart is normal in size. There is no pericardial effusion. There is no lymphadenopathy in the chest.
Bones and soft tissues:
No acute osseous abnormalities are identified.
Upper abdomen:
Evaluation of the upper abdomen is limited by technique. The visualized upper abdomen is unremarkable.

32.2 Stakeholders

Cardiothoracic radiologists, general radiologists, radiology residents and fellows, and emergency medicine physicians and providers.

32.3 Pearls

- CT pulmonary angiography (CTPA) examinations have largely supplanted ventilation-perfusion scans for the assessment of pulmonary embolism (▶ Fig. 32.1). Advantages of CTPA include wide availability, rapid acquisition, and high positive predictive value.
- Several studies have demonstrated that CTPA reports are more complete and accurate when disease-specific templates are used in clinical workflows.
- In one study evaluating the inclusion of elements outlined in the RSNA template for CTPA studies, only 16% of reports contained all important elements. The most common elements not

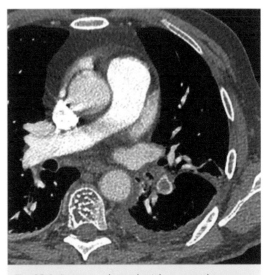

Fig. 32.1 Contrast-enhanced axial computed tomography (CT) pulmonary angiography demonstrates a central filling defect in a left lower lobe segmental pulmonary artery compatible with pulmonary embolus.

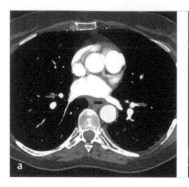
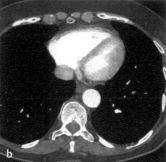

Fig. 32.2 **(a)** Contrast-enhanced axial computed tomography (CT) pulmonary angiography shows filling defects in bilateral lower lobe subsegmental pulmonary arteries compatible with pulmonary emboli. **(b)** CT of the same patient at the level of the heart demonstrates dilatation of the right ventricle with a right ventricle-to-left ventricle ratio > 0.9, compatible with right heart strain.

included in the free-form reports included the technical quality of the study and the presence of potential complications such as right heart strain and pulmonary infarction.[1]

- In another study, the institution of a disease-specific template increased the completeness of CTPA reports from 69 to 96%.[2]
- The first parameter that should be assessed on all CTPA examinations is the *technical quality* (or how adequately the pulmonary arteries are opacified with intravenous contrast).
- If emboli are present, additional details such as the *laterality, specific location within the pulmonary arterial tree, chronicity, and multiplicity* should be included.
- Potential complications of pulmonary embolism such *as right heart strain and pulmonary infarction* should be noted. Right heart strain can be assessed qualitatively and quantitatively. *Qualitative* findings suggestive of *right heart strain* include right ventricular enlargement, flattening of the interventricular septum, bowing of the interventricular septum toward the left ventricle, enlargement of the pulmonary trunk, reflux of contrast into the inferior vena cava, a dilated azygous venous system, and dilated hepatic veins with or without reflux of contrast.
- The primary *quantitative* method of assessing *right heart strain* is the calculation of the right ventricle-to-left ventricle ratio, which is typically measured on axial CT images (▸ Fig. 32.2). A right ventricle-to-left ventricle diameter ratio > 0.9 is suggestive of right heart strain.
- *Pulmonary infarction* classically manifests as a peripheral wedge-shaped opacity that may be consolidative, ground-glass, or a combination

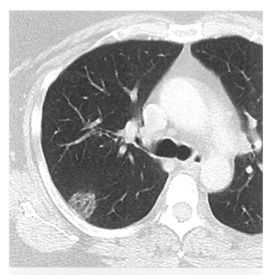

Fig. 32.3 Contrast-enhanced axial computed tomography (CT) pulmonary angiography (lung windows) of a patient with bilateral pulmonary emboli (not shown) demonstrates a nodular opacity in the right lower lobe that is predominantly ground-glass in attenuation, suggestive of pulmonary infarction.

(▸ Fig. 32.3). Pulmonary hemorrhage may be present in the adjacent lung parenchyma.

References

[1] Carter BW, Steele JR, Sun J, Wu CC. Analysis of the completeness and clarity of free-form radiology dictations for the reporting of pulmonary embolism. J Am Coll Radiol. 2017; 14 (12):1556–1559

[2] Chung JH, Landeras L, Haas K, Liu P, Liu L, MacMahon H. The value of a disease-specific template and an IT-based quality tracking system in pulmonary embolism CT angiography. J Am Coll Radiol. 2018; 15(7):988–992

33 Tracheobronchomalacia

Daniela M. Tridente and Diana Litmanovich

33.1 Template

Findings:
Dynamic CT of the airways:
- Tracheal shape in end-inspiration: [normal/stenotic/saber sheath/post tracheoplasty/other]
- Tracheal shape in dynamic expiration: [normal/stenotic/lunate/other]
- Tracheal wall thickness: [normal/thickened]—(if thickened) [circumferential/anterior wall]

Tracheal collapsibility:
1 cm above the aortic arch (coronal × sagittal diameters; area)
- Inspiration: [ ] × [ ] mm, [ ] mm^2
- Expiration: [ ] × [ ] mm, [ ] mm^2
- Collapsibility index (CI): (I–E)/I × 100 = [ ]% decrease in the tracheal area

1 cm above the carina (coronal × sagittal diameters; area)
- Inspiration: [ ] × [ ] mm, [ ] mm^2
- Expiration: [ ] × [ ] mm, [ ] mm^2
- Collapsibility index (CI): (I – E)/I × 100 = [ ]% decrease in the tracheal area

(Complete following section if there is an area with collapsibility higher than either 1 cm above the aortic arch or 1 cm above the carina)
Level of most severe tracheal collapse (coronal × sagittal diameters; area)
- Anatomical level: [ ] cm above the carina
- Inspiration: [ ] × [ ] mm, [ ] mm^2
- Expiration: [ ] × [ ]mm, [ ] mm^2
- Collapsibility index (CI): (I – E)/I × 100 = [ ]% decrease in the tracheal area

Focal narrowing or stricture: [absent/present]
(if absent, please delete dedicated section below)
Proximal margin at end-inspiration: [ ] mm below vocal cords
Length at end-inspiration: [ ] mm
Level of most severe narrowing (coronal × sagittal diameters; area)
- Inspiration: [ ] × [ ] mm, [ ] mm^2
- Expiration: [ ] × [ ] mm, [ ] mm^2

Bronchi collapsibility:
Right main bronchus, at the level of maximum collapse
- Inspiration: [ ] mm
- Expiration: [ ] mm
- Collapsibility index (CI): (I – E)/I × 100 = [ ]% decrease in the bronchial area

Left main bronchus, at the level of maximum collapse
- Inspiration: [ ] mm
- Expiration: [ ] mm
- Collapsibility index (CI): (I – E)/I × 100 = [ ]% decrease in the bronchial area

Air trapping: [none/mild/moderate/severe]
Impression:
- No/evidence of tracheomalacia (% collapse)
- No/evidence of bronchomalacia (% collapse)
- No/evidence of focal tracheal narrowing
- [Other findings]

33.2 Stakeholders

Cardiothoracic radiologists, interventional pulmonologists, pulmonologists, thoracic surgeons, and
primary care physicians.

33.3 Pearls

- Tracheobronchomalacia (TBM) is defined as
  reduction of the airway lumen area by more
  than 70% during forced expiration. There are
  multiple known causes for TBM (► Fig. 33.1)
  such as relapsing polychondritis, prolonged
  intubation trauma, or congenital connective
  tissue disorders; however, it can also be
  idiopathic.
- Multidetector computed tomography (MDCT) is
  a reliable noninvasive method to diagnose TBM.
  Its accuracy is comparable to bronchoscopy, the

historical reference standard for diagnosis of
TBM. CT is useful for both initial diagnosis and
follow-up.
- Imaging acquisition comprises two different
  phases: end-inspiratory (EI) phase (reflecting
  total lung capacity and maximum airway size)
  and dynamic expiratory (DE) phase, acquired
  during forced expiration (► Fig. 33.2).
- The tracheal wall is usually visible as 1- to 3-mm
  soft tissue density line, with smooth inner and
  outer margins. The posterior wall is typically
  thinner than the anterior and lateral walls.
  Calcification of the cartilage in the anterior and
  lateral tracheal wall is a normal sign of aging,
  especially in women. Thickening of the airway
  wall and its location are important for diagnosis
  of airway pathologies. Disorders that involve
  cartilage would spare the posterior membrane
  (for example, relapsing polychondritis) as

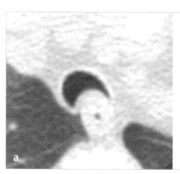
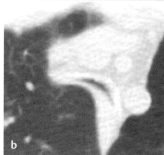

Fig. 33.1 Axial noncontrast-enhanced multidetector computed tomography (MDCT) images of the chest demonstrating (a) mild (70%) and (b) severe (90%) tracheal collapsibility during dynamic expiration.

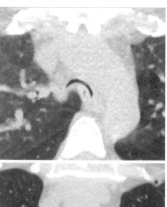
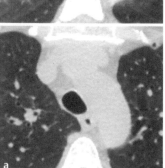
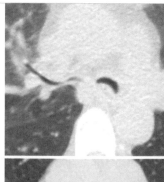
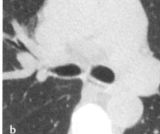

Fig. 33.2 Severe (a) tracheomalacia (91%) and (b) right bronchomalacia (88%) on standard end-inspiration (superior) and dynamic expiration (inferior) axial images.

opposed to inflammatory conditions, such as granulomatous polyangiitis and sarcoidosis, which would cause circumferential thickening.

- On axial CT images at end-inspiration the normal tracheal lumen (► Fig. 33.3a) is most commonly round or slightly oval in shape, with coronal-to-sagittal diameter ratio close to 1. Common abnormal tracheal shapes are lunate and saber-sheath. Lunate (► Fig. 33.3b) configuration refers to increased coronal diameter with relative narrowing of the sagittal diameter (coronal:sagittal diameter > 1). Saber-sheath trachea (► Fig. 33.3c), frequently seen in patients with chronic obstructive pulmonary disease (COPD), is characterized by marked coronal diameter narrowing and accentuation of the sagittal diameter (coronal:sagittal diameter < 1). Both shapes are frequently associated with tracheomalacia.

- After tracheobronchoplasty, a surgical procedure done to augment the posterior wall of the trachea and bronchi in order to decrease expiratory collapsibility, the trachea acquires an inverted D shape (► Fig. 33.3d).

- Cross-sectional area measurements should be performed consistently at predetermined levels (► Fig. 33.4). The widely accepted and recommended levels are: 1 cm above the aortic arch, 1 cm above the carina, and 1 cm below the carina for both left and right main bronchi.

- Airway lumen measurements should be performed in lung windows in the true transverse plane of the airway determined with multiplanar reconstructions and defined as perpendicular to the long axis of the airway. These measurements provide best diagnostic accuracy (► Fig. 33.5).

- Collapsibility index is defined as the difference between the cross-sectional areas of end-inspiration and forced expiration divided by that of end-inspiration, times a 100 (percentage).

- Though there is no universal classification of severity, reduction of lumen in more than 90% is considered severe disease and a potential threshold for plication of the membranous wall of the trachea (or tracheobronchoplasty) in patients with severe symptoms.

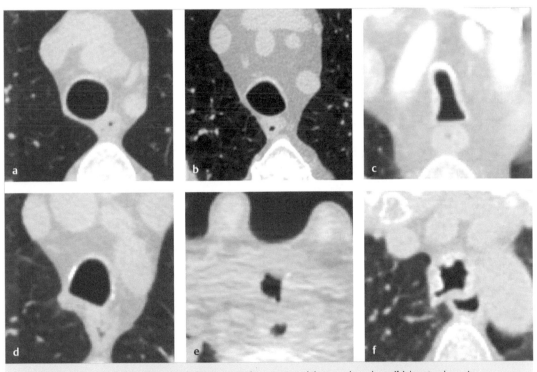

Fig. 33.3 Examples of different tracheal shapes at end-inspiration: (a) normal trachea; (b) lunate shape in tracheomalacia; (c) saber-sheath trachea in chronic obstructive pulmonary disease (COPD); (d) post-tracheoplasty; (e) stenotic trachea due to prolonged intubation; (f) irregular trachea with polyps in tracheobronchopathia osteochondroplastica.

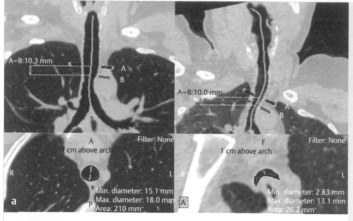

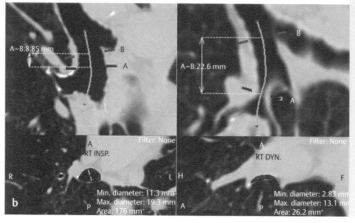

Fig. 33.4 Automatic measurement process using airway centerline to create true transverse images perpendicular to the long axis of the airway for measuring cross-sectional areas at predetermined levels, for example **(a)** 1 cm above aortic arch in the trachea and **(b)** 1 cm below the carina in the right main bronchus.

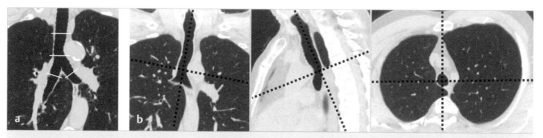

Fig. 33.5 Coronal image **(a)** demonstrates the predetermined levels for assessment of tracheobronchial collapsibility. Coronal, sagittal, and axial images **(b)** demonstrate the process of double-oblique reconstruction to create a true transverse plane to measure the cross-sectional area at a given level.

- Isolated complete collapse of the bronchus intermedius should not raise the possibility of bronchomalacia since it has been found in a significant number of healthy individuals.
- An alternative way to create a true transverse plane of the airway is by applying automatic curved centerline with subsequent perpendicular axial planes of the predetermined levels (▶ Fig. 33.4).

- When using automated reconstruction methods, the diameters provided reflect the maximum and minimum diameters of the airway area which usually correspond closely to the coronal and sagittal diameters, respectively.
- Standardization of the measured segments is key to ensure analytical accuracy, allowing for better consistency when comparing studies, especially after surgical interventions.

Suggested Readings

Bezuidenhout, AF, Boiselle, PM, Heidinger, BH, Alape, D, Buitrago, DH, Majid, A, Gangadharan, SP, Litmanovich, DE. Longitudinal follow-up of patients with tracheobronchomalacia after undergoing tracheobronchoplasty: CT findings and clinical correlation. J Thorac Imaging. 2019; 34(4):278–283

Ciet P, Boiselle PM, Michaud G, O'Donnell C, Litmanovich DE. Optimal imaging protocol for measuring dynamic expiratory collapse of the central airways. Clin Radiol. 2016; 71(1):e49–e55

Heidinger BH, Occhipinti M, Eisenberg RL, Bankier AA. Imaging of large airways disorders. AJR Am J Roentgenol. 2015; 205(1): 41–56

Lee EY, Litmanovich D, Boiselle PM. Multidetector CT evaluation of tracheobronchomalacia. Radiol Clin North Am. 2009; 47(2): 261–269

Litmanovich D, O'Donnell CR, Bankier AA, et al. Bronchial collapsibility at forced expiration in healthy volunteers: assessment with multidetector CT. Radiology. 2010; 257(2):560–567

O'Donnell CR, Bankier AA, O'Donnell DH, Loring SH, Boiselle PM. Static end-expiratory and dynamic forced expiratory tracheal collapse in COPD. Clin Radiol. 2014; 69(4):357–362

34 Fibrotic Lung Disease

Mary Frances Croake, Hakan Sahin, and Katherine Kaproth-Joslin

34.1 Template

Lungs and distal airways:
Findings related to pulmonary fibrosis:
- Zonal distribution: cranial-caudal distribution: [upper lung predominant/mid-lung predominant/lower lung predominant/diffuse]; axial distribution: [central/peripheral/peripheral with subpleural sparing/diffuse]; [free text]
- Honeycombing: [none/mild/moderate/severe]; [free text]
- Traction bronchiectasis: [none/mild/moderate/severe]; [free text]
- Reticulation: [none/mild/moderate/severe]; [free text]

Findings not related to pulmonary fibrosis:
- Ground-glass opacity: [none/mild/moderate/severe]; [free text]
- Air-trapping: [none/mild/moderate/severe]; [free text]
- Nodules: [present/absent]; if present: density: [solid/semisolid/ground-glass]; pattern of distribution: [random/centrilobular/perilymphatic]; zonal distribution: [upper lung predominant/mid-lung predominant/lower lung predominant/diffuse]; [free text description, size, and location]
- Cysts/Consolidation: [present/absent]; [free text description/location]
- Emphysema: [none/mild/moderate/severe]; If present type [paraseptal/centrilobular/panlobular/mixed]; [free text]
- Other lung findings: [free text]

Mediastinum and lymph nodes:
- Esophagus: dilation: [present/absent]; wall thickening: [present/absent]; hiatal hernia: [present/absent]; [free text]
- Lymph nodes: lymphadenopathy: [present/absent], if present [example location (s)] [size] mm; calcifications: [present/absent]; [free text]

Cardiovascular structures:
- Pulmonary artery: main size [ ] cm; [free text]
- Aorta: ascending size [ ] cm; calcifications: [none/mild/moderate/severe]; [free text]
- Coronary calcifications: [none/mild/moderate/severe]; [free text]
- Cardiac chambers: [chambers] are [normal/mildly enlarged/moderately enlarged/severely enlarged]; [free text]
- Pericardium is [normal/thickened] [with/without effusion]; [free text]

Pleura and pleural space: [apical pleural thickening present/absent]; [pleural fluid collection present/absent]; [free text]
Impression:
- Impression related to pulmonary fibrosis: [free text]
- Overall change since prior: [unchanged/increased when compared to prior/decreased when compared with prior imaging/no prior imaging available for comparison]
- Imaging pattern of pulmonary fibrosis: [typical UIP CT pattern/probable UIP CT pattern/CT pattern indeterminate for UIP/CT features most consistent with non-IPF diagnosis]
- [Other impressionable findings]

Table 34.1 Diagnostic categories of UIP on CT

	Typical UIP CT pattern	Probable UIP CT pattern	CT pattern indeterminate for UIP	CT features most consistent with non-IPF diagnosis
CT distribution	Basal (occasionally diffuse) and subpleural predominant Distribution is often heterogeneous	Basal and subpleural predominant. Distribution is often heterogeneous	Variable or diffuse	Upper or mid-lung predominant fibrosis Peribronchovascular predominance with subpleural sparing
CT features	Honeycombing Reticular pattern with peripheral traction bronchiectasis or bronchiolectasis[a] Absence of features to suggest an alternative diagnosis	Reticular pattern with peripheral traction bronchiectasis or bronchiolectasis[a] Honeycombing is absent	Evidence of fibrosis with some inconspicuous features suggestive of non-UIP pattern[a]	Any of the following: Predominant consolidation Extensive pure ground-glass opacity (without acute exacerbation) Extensive mosaic attenuation with extensive sharply defined lobular air trapping on expiration Diffuse nodules or cysts

Abbreviations: CT, computed tomography; IPF, idiopathic pulmonary fibrosis; UIP, usual interstitial pneumonia.
[a]Reticular pattern is superimposed on ground glass opacity, and in these cases is usually fibrotic. Pure ground glass opacity however would be against the diagnosis of UIP/IPF and would suggest acute exacerbation, hypersensitivity pneumonitis or other conditions. (Reproduced with permission of Lynch DA, Sverzellati N, Travis WD, et al. Diagnostic criteria for idiopathic pulmonary fibrosis: a Fleischner Society White Paper. Lancet Respir Med. Elsevier; 2018; 6(2):138–153.)

34.2 Stakeholders

Pulmonologist, thoracic surgeon, interventional radiologist, radiologist, and pathologist. Given the complexity and often confounding clinical picture of interstitial lung disease, the radiologist plays a central role in identifying patterns of lung disease, synthesizing the clinical data, and relaying results in a clear and concise language that can be easily integrated by the pulmonologist, thoracic surgeon, interventional radiologist, and pathologist to determine if biopsy is necessary and to guide the management and treatment options.

34.3 Pearls

- Imaging quality:
  - Volumetric acquisition, thin section (< 2 mm), high spatial resolution reconstructions, and images obtained at full inspiration.
  - Prone imaging is beneficial, particularly when there is dependent opacification which can mimic subtle disease.
  - Expiratory imaging is often necessary to identify air-trapping (which is an atypical feature for usual interstitial pneumonia (UIP) and may be helpful in differentiating this condition from chronic hypersensitivity pneumonitis (HP).

- In the setting of pulmonary fibrosis, the radiologist must report whether a UIP pattern is present and the interpreter's confidence level. Diagnostic categories of UIP patterns on computed tomography (CT) include: typical, probable, indeterminate, and non–idiopathic pulmonary fibrosis (non-IPF) diagnosis (▶ Table 34.1).
- Identification of typical and probable UIP pattern on CT supports a diagnosis of IPF in the appropriate clinical setting, delineated by the presence or absence of honeycombing, respectively.
- Typical UIP features include: basal and subpleural predominant distribution with honeycombing, peripheral reticular pattern, and traction bronchiectasis (▶ Fig. 34.1).
- Honeycombing is defined as clustered, thick-walled, cystic spaces of similar diameters measuring 3 to 5 mm with at least two to three contiguous subpleural layers. Presence of honeycombing suggests worse prognosis.
- Traction bronchiectasis is a hallmark of lung fibrosis and a prognostic marker.
- A reticular pattern is characterized by a network of fine lines (typically irregularly spaced with a mixture of thick and thin lines in UIP).
- Emphysema can be a confounding factor in patients with an UIP pattern on CT. The extent

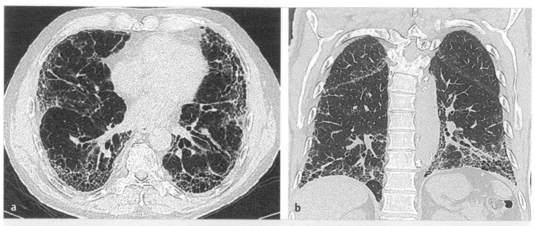

Fig. 34.1 (a, b) Axial and coronal images demonstrate typical usual interstitial pneumonia (UIP) computed tomography (CT) pattern with a lower lung predominant craniocaudal distribution, peripheral axial distribution of reticulation, and subpleural involvement. This is associated with traction bronchiectasis and honeycombing.

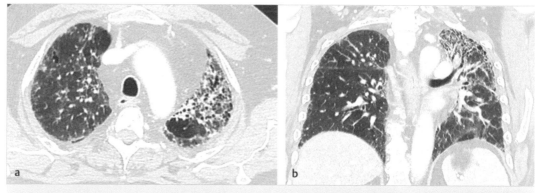

Fig. 34.2 (a, b) Axial and coronal computed tomography (CT) image demonstrates CT features most consistent with non–idiopathic pulmonary fibrosis (non-IPF) diagnosis with an upper lung predominant craniocaudal distribution, primarily peripheral axial reticulation, and subpleural involvement. This is associated with traction bronchiectasis and honeycombing. These findings favor a diagnosis of chronic hypersensitivity pneumonitis (HP).

and relative severity should be reported as it influences patient management and prognosis.

- The presence of mosaic attenuation and air trapping are helpful in distinguishing UIP from chronic HP.
- Typical features of chronic HP include upper or mid-lung distribution, profuse centrilobular nodules, mosaic attenuation, and air trapping (▶ Fig. 34.2).
- Pleural effusion, esophageal dilation, or pericardial abnormality in a patient with pulmonary fibrosis regardless of confidence of UIP pattern should raise the possibility of underlying connective tissue disease.

- Hiatal hernia along with esophageal thickening/dilation is an important finding, as chronic aspiration is an underreported but common cause of fibrosis involving the basilar lungs.
- The presence of subpleural sparring and predominant ground-glass opacities should lead to consideration of nonspecific interstitial pneumonia (NSIP). Typical features of NSIP include: lower lobe distribution, predominant patchy ground-glass opacities, fine reticular pattern with subpleural sparring (▶ Fig. 34.3).
- Cardiac chamber and pulmonary arterial size should be reported as the presence of pulmonary hypertension can be an important prognostic factor.

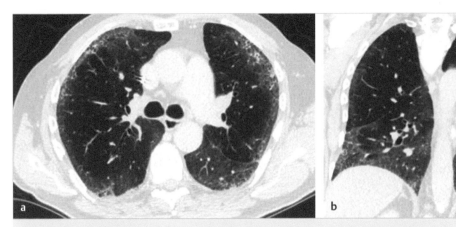

Fig. 34.3 (a, b) Axial and coronal computed tomography (CT) images demonstrate CT features most consistent with non–idiopathic pulmonary fibrosis (non-IPF) diagnosis with a diffuse craniocaudal distribution and slight basal predominance, primarily peripheral reticulation and ground-glass opacity, and evidence of relative subpleural sparing. Note the lack of honeycombing and significant traction bronchiectasis. These findings favor a diagnosis of nonspecific interstitial pneumonia (NSIP).

- Lymphadenopathy and pulmonary nodules are common findings with underlying ILD; however, an asymmetrically growing nodule or lymph node should be critically considered, as the risk of developing malignancy is elevated in this patient population.

Suggested Readings

Chung JH, Chawla A, Peljto AL, et al. CT scan findings of probable usual interstitial pneumonitis have a high predictive value for histologic usual interstitial pneumonitis. Chest. 2015; 147 (2):450–459

Chung JH, Lynch DA. The value of a multidisciplinary approach to the diagnosis of usual interstitial pneumonitis and idiopathic pulmonary fibrosis: radiology, pathology, and clinical correlation. AJR Am J Roentgenol. 2016; 206(3):463–471

Ferguson EC, Berkowitz EA. Lung CT: part 2, the interstitial pneumonias—clinical, histologic, and CT manifestations. AJR Am J Roentgenol. 2012; 199(4):W464–76

Lynch DA, Sverzellati N, Travis WD, et al. Diagnostic criteria for idiopathic pulmonary fibrosis: a Fleischner Society White Paper. Lancet Respir Med. 2018; 6(2):138–153

Raghu G, Remy-Jardin M, Myers JL, et al. American Thoracic Society, European Respiratory Society, Japanese Respiratory Society, and Latin American Thoracic Society. Diagnosis of idiopathic pulmonary fibrosis: an official ATS/ERS/JRS/ALAT clinical practice guideline. Am J Respir Crit Care Med. 2018; 198(5):e44–e68

35 Pulmonary Hypertension CTPA

Seth Kligerman

35.1 Template

Pulmonary arteries:

Bolus: [good/suboptimal but adequate/nondiagnostic]. If nondiagnostic, state lobes or segments where diagnostic is not possible

Respiratory motion: [none/mild/moderate/severe]. If moderate or severe, state levels that are nondiagnostic due to motion

Main pulmonary artery diameter: [ ] cm; aorta diameter: [ ] cm; aorta to PA ratio: [ ]

Right ventricle (RV): [normal/abnormal]. If abnormal, state whether the RV is dilated or hypertrophied; ratio of right ventricle-to-left ventricle axial diameter: [ ]

Peripheral pulmonary arteries: [normal/(focally or diffusely) enlarged and/or tortuous/(focally or diffusely) attenuated]

Filling defects: [none/present]. If present, specify distribution and whether PE appears acute, chronic, or acute superimposed on chronic

Iodine map (if dual energy is performed): [normal/abnormal]. If abnormal, state segmental areas of hypo-perfusion and hyperperfusion and whether they correspond to location of pulmonary emboli and enlarged pulmonary artery branches, respectively

Mediastinum:

Thyroid and thoracic inlet: [normal]

Lymph nodes: [normal]. If enlarged, state distribution and short-axis diameter

Esophagus: [normal/abnormal]

Other cardiovascular:

Carefully assess for undiagnosed congenital heart disease as a cause of pulmonary hypertension (atrial septal defect, ventricular septal defect, PAPVR, etc)

Atherosclerotic disease: [none/mild/moderate/severe] involving the [aorta/coronary arteries/aorta and coronary arteries]

Left ventricle: [normal/abnormal]. If abnormal, state findings

Arch vessels and visualized arteries: [normal/abnormal]

Atrial size: [normal/enlarged]. Systemic veins: [normal/abnormal]

State whether the IVC and/or SVC are dilated. Pericardium: [normal/abnormal]

Lungs:

Trachea and large airways: [normal/abnormal]. If abnormal, state whether large airways are thickened, bronchiectatic, or stenotic

Parenchyma: [normal/abnormal]. If abnormal, discuss

- Nodules: [absent/present]. If present, discuss location, size, and distribution
- Mosaicism: [absent/present]. If present, discuss distribution (lobe) and extent of mosaicism (lobular, subsegmental, segmental, lobar, etc.). Discuss whether vessels are normal or small in size in hypoattenuated areas and whether vessels are large in size in hyperattenuated areas (commonly seen in patients with chronic thromboembolic disease pulmonary hypertension [CTEPH]). Discuss the presence of periarteriolar blushing if present (commonly seen in patients with pulmonary arterial hypertension)
- Emphysema: [absent/present]. If present, trace, mild, moderate, confluent, advanced destructive
- Interstitial abnormality: [absent/present]. If present, discuss location, presence, and degree or septal thickening, reticulation, scarring, etc

Other: [none]

Pleura:

[Normal/abnormal]. If abnormal, state whether there are pleural effusions (mild, moderate, severe), pleural thickening, pleural plaques, or other abnormality

Superior abdomen:
[Normal/abnormal]. Hepatic veins are [normal/dilated]
Bones and soft tissues:
[Normal/abnormal]

Table 35.1 Pulmonary arterial hypertension groups 1–5 as classified by WHO[1]

Pulmonary arterial hypertension (group 1)	PHTN due to left heart disease (group 2)	PHTN due to lung disease (group 3)	Chronic thromboembolic pulmonary hypertension (group 4)	PHTN with unclear or multifactorial mechanisms (group 5)
Idiopathic PAH	Left ventricular systolic dysfunction	Chronic obstructive pulmonary disease (COPD)		Hematologic disorders
Heritable 1. BMPR2 (80%) 2. ALK 1 3. Endoglin 4. SMAD 1,4,9	Left ventricular diastolic dysfunction	Interstitial lung disease		Systemic disorders that have lung involvement: 1. Sarcoidosis 2. Pulmonary Langerhans cell histiocytosis 3. Vasculitis
Drug and toxin induced: 1. Amphetamines and methamphetamines 2. Cocaine 3. Fen-Phen	Valvular heart disease	Sleep apnea		Metabolic disorders
Associated with systemic disease: 1. Connective tissue disease 2. HIV infection 3. Portal hypertension 4. Congenital heart disease	Left heart inflow and outflow obstruction not due to valvular or congenital heart disease	Development lung abnormalities		Other diseases not well classified elsewhere
Pulmonary veno-occlusive disease/pulmonary capillary hemangiomatosis		Alveolar hypoventilation disorders		

Abbreviations: PAH, pulmonary arterial hypertension; PHTN, pulmonary hypertension.

35.2 Stakeholders

Pulmonologists and thoracic surgeons.

35.3 Pearls

- There are numerous causes of pulmonary hypertension (PH) which are classified as group 1–5 according to WHO (▶ Table 35.1).
- In many cases of PH, the pulmonary artery is enlarged. While various numbers have been suggested as a cutoff for maximum pulmonary artery size, this method is not accurate. A better measurement is to compare the diameter of the aorta to the pulmonary artery. In general, when the pulmonary artery is larger than the aorta, PH can be suggested.
- The imaging features of PH vary depending on the cause. In more advanced cases, the central pulmonary arteries are enlarged, the right ventricle is hypertrophied, the interventricular septum can be flattened, and the right atrium is dilated.
- While the findings in the central pulmonary arteries and heart may be similar among causes of PH, the appearance of the peripheral vessels and pulmonary parenchyma may help to differentiate etiologies.

- Pulmonary arterial hypertension (PAH) is classified as group 1 (▶ Table 35.1) and may be idiopathic or secondary. The main treatment for PAH is with medical therapy. When medical therapy fails, double lung transplantation is recommended with heart-lung transplantation reserved to those with severe right ventricular dysfunction or congenital heart disease.[2]
- The imaging manifestations of PAH can vary but the pulmonary parenchyma often ill-defined centrilobular or periarteriolar ground-glass opacity and/or nodules[3] (▶ Fig. 35.1). This can lead to a mosaic pattern of attenuation without the segmental or subsegmental distribution seen in chronic thromboembolic disease pulmonary hypertension (CTEPH). The peripheral vessels can demonstrate a combination of both tortuous vessels and/or abrupt decrease in caliber near the periphery of the lung.[4]
- Pulmonary veno-occlusive disease (PVOD) and pulmonary capillary hemangiomatosis (PCH), which are classified within group 1, are thought to represent a continuum of arterial, capillary, and vein involvement in PAH. Recently, PVOD and PCH have been reclassified as a single entity titled "PAH with over features of venous/capillary involvement."[5] Compared to other causes of PAH, PAH with over features of venous/capillary involvement should be suspected in

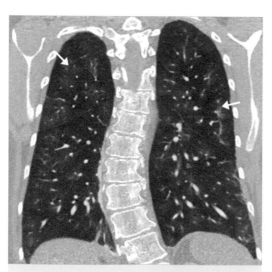

Fig. 35.1 Coronal computed tomography (CT) image of a 23-year-old woman with pulmonary arterial hypertension (PAH) shows nodular periarteriolar ground-glass opacities throughout the lungs (*white arrows*). This finding is common in patients with PAH but atypical in other findings of pulmonary hypertension.

patients with PH with prominent septal thickening and/or centrilobular ground-glass nodules.[3,6] Left ventricular function in these patients is often normal, which helps in differentiating from pulmonary edema.

- PH due to left heart disease is classified as group 2 and is secondary to left ventricular systolic or diastolic failure, severe left-sided valvular disease, and congenital heart disease. While some findings associated with group 2 disease such as left ventricular dilation can be assessed with nongated CT pulmonary angiography, this diagnosis is usually made with echocardiography, cardiac magnetic resonance imaging (MRI), or ECG-gated cardiac CT angiography.
- Patients with group 3 PH have PH secondary to lung disease and/or chronic hypoxia. Most commonly, this is seen in patients with severe COPD.[7] Therefore, one should assess the parenchyma for findings of smoking-related lung disease most notably emphysema and bronchial wall thickening. Pulmonary fibrosis is another common cause of group 3 PH, and findings of reticulation, traction bronchiectasis, volume loss, and honeycombing should be reported. Although obstructive sleep apnea can be seen in a variety of patients, the findings of PH in an obese patient may suggest this diagnosis.
- While most forms of PH are treated medically, CTEPH, classified as group 4, is the only form where surgery (pulmonary thromboendarterectomy) is the primary therapy.[8] Therefore, differentiation between CTEPH and other forms of pulmonary hypertension is very important
- CTEPH has various imaging appearances. Most commonly, there is adherent thrombus along the walls of the pulmonary arteries. Compared to acute PE where occluded vessels are expanded, in CTEPH the occluded arteries are contracted due to scarring and contraction or organized thrombus. Other findings include abrupt cutoff or decrease in caliber of vessels. Unlike PAH where one sees diffuse peripheral pruning of the vasculature, the abrupt vascular cutoffs in CTEPH are variable and occur throughout the pulmonary artery tree. Webs are secondary to partial recanalization of thrombus and dilated bronchial arteries are also common findings.[9]
- Parenchymal findings in CTEPH are often characteristic with lobar, segmental, or subsegmental areas of hypoperfusion

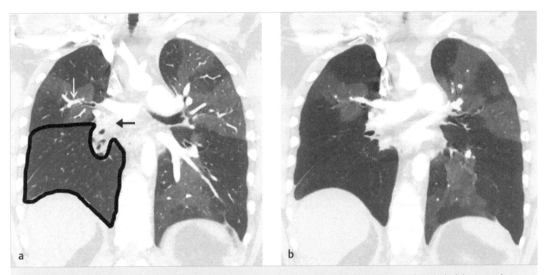

Fig. 35.2 25-year-old man with chronic thromboembolic disease pulmonary hypertension (CTEPH). **(a)** Coronal multiplanar reformat (MPR) shows occlusion of the interlobar pulmonary artery (*black arrow*) as well as numerous other segmental and subsegmental branches. The areas distal to the interlobar occlusion (*black outline*) is hypoattenuated due to lack of blood flow. The areas with unobstructed vessels demonstrate compensatory hyperperfusion (*white outline*) with dilation of the associated pulmonary artery branches (*white arrows*). **(b)** 4mm thick minimum intensity projection image (MinIP) nicely demonstrates this mosaic perfusion.

corresponding to the vascular distribution of vascular thrombosis. In severe cases, there are often areas of segmental and subsegmental hyperattenuation due to hyperperfusion from enlarged, tortuous vessels[3] (▶ Fig. 35.2).

- Group 5 pulmonary hypertension represents variable diseases that do not fit into other categories. Except for sarcoidosis, most are difficult to diagnose on CT pulmonary angiography (CTPA).

References

[1] Galiè N, McLaughlin VV, Rubin LJ, Simonneau G. An overview of the 6th World Symposium on Pulmonary Hypertension. Eur Respir J. 2019; 53(1)

[2] Lordan JL, Corris PA. Pulmonary arterial hypertension and lung transplantation. Expert Rev Respir Med. 2011; 5 (3):441–454

[3] Kligerman SJ, Henry T, Lin CT, Franks TJ, Galvin JR. Mosaic attenuation: etiology, methods of differentiation, and pitfalls. Radiographics. 2015; 35(5):1360–1380

[4] Grosse C, Grosse A. CT findings in diseases associated with pulmonary hypertension: a current review. Radiographics. 2010; 30(7):1753–1777

[5] Simonneau G, Montani D, Celermajer DS, et al. Haemodynamic definitions and updated clinical classification of pulmonary hypertension. Eur Respir J. 2019; 53(1):1801913

[6] Frazier AA, Franks TJ, Mohammed TL, Ozbudak IH, Galvin JR. From the archives of the AFIP: pulmonary veno-occlusive disease and pulmonary capillary hemangiomatosis. Radiographics. 2007; 27(3):867–882

[7] Nathan SD, Barbera JA, Gaine SP, et al. Pulmonary hypertension in chronic lung disease and hypoxia. Eur Respir J. 2019; 53(1):1801914

[8] Kim NH, Delcroix M, Jenkins DP, et al. Chronic thromboembolic pulmonary hypertension. J Am Coll Cardiol. 2013; 62 (25) Suppl:D92–D99

[9] Gopalan D, Delcroix M, Held M. Diagnosis of chronic thromboembolic pulmonary hypertension. Eur Respir Rev. 2017; 26(143):160108

36 Chronic Obstructive Pulmonary Disease

David A. Lynch

36.1 Template

Lung volumes: [increased/decreased/normal]
Parenchymal emphysema: [present/absent]
- Parenchymal emphysema grade: [trace centrilobular/mild centrilobular/moderate centrilobular/ confluent/advanced destructive
- Parenchymal emphysema distribution: [upper lung predominant/lower lung predominant/mid-lung predominant/diffuse]

Paraseptal emphysema: [present/absent]
- Paraseptal emphysema grade: [mild/substantial]
- Large bullae (> 5 cm): [present/absent]

Bronchial wall thickening: [present/absent]
Centrilobular nodularity: [present/absent]
Expiratory air trapping: [absent/present only in emphysematous areas/present in non-emphysematous regions]
Associated features:
Fissural completeness (in patients with moderate or severe emphysema):
- Right major fissure: [complete (> 90%)/incomplete]
- Right minor fissure: [complete (> 90%)/incomplete]
- Left major fissure: [complete (> 90%)/incomplete]

Mucoid impaction: [present/absent]
Mucoid impaction location: [segmental/subsegmental/small bronchi]
Bronchiectasis: [present/absent]
Main pulmonary artery: [dilated/not dilated]

36.2 Stakeholders

Pulmonologists, interventional pulmonologists, and surgeons.

36.3 Pearls

- Chronic obstructive pulmonary disease (COPD) is the fourth commonest cause of death in the United States, and a major cause of disability.
- It is defined on the basis of airflow obstruction: ratio of forced expiratory volume in 1 second to forced vital capacity (FEV1/FVC) < 0.70. However, individuals who do meet criteria for obstruction may also have important morbidity and mortality.
- COPD is morphologically heterogenous: some individuals with COPD have predominant emphysema (▶ Fig. 36.1), others have predominant airway wall thickening, and some have small airways disease with expiratory air

trapping. Most have some combination of these components, all of which may contribute to mortality.
- The grade of parenchymal emphysema is an independent risk factor for mortality.
- Paraseptal emphysema is a risk factor for pneumothorax.
- Expiratory air trapping provides the best correlation with airflow obstruction.
- Bronchial wall thickening is associated with potentially reversible airflow obstruction and with increased risk of exacerbations.
- When emphysema and/or COPD is identified in nonsmokers, potential causes may include secondhand smoke, alpha-1 antitrypsin deficiency (lower lobe panlobular emphysema), pneumoconiosis, hypersensitivity pneumonitis, and vasculitis.
- Fissural completeness is important in patients with moderate or advanced emphysema, to

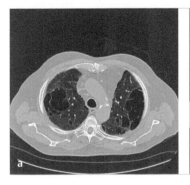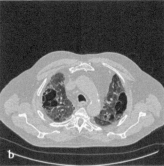

Fig. 36.1 Inspiratory axial image **(a)** from noncontrast chest computed tomography (CT) shows a combination of paraseptal and centrilobular emphysema, which is accentuated on expiration **(b)**.

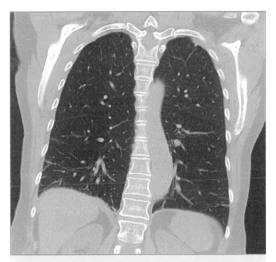

Fig. 36.2 Coronal image from noncontrast chest computed tomography (CT) shows incomplete major fissures medially.

placement or lung volume reduction surgery (▶ Fig. 36.2).

Suggested Readings

Han MK, Kazerooni EA, Lynch DA, et al. COPDGene Investigators. Chronic obstructive pulmonary disease exacerbations in the COPDGene study: associated radiologic phenotypes. Radiology. 2011; 261(1):274–282

Lynch DA, Moore CM, Wilson C, et al. Genetic Epidemiology of COPD (COPDGene) Investigators. CT-based visual classification of emphysema: association with mortality in the COPDGene study. Radiology. 2018; 288(3):859–866

Lynch DA, Sverzellati N, Travis WD, et al. Diagnostic criteria for idiopathic pulmonary fibrosis: a Fleischner Society White Paper. Lancet Respir Med. 2017

Regan EA, Lynch DA, Curran-Everett D, et al. Genetic Epidemiology of COPD (COPDGene) Investigators. Clinical and radiologic disease in smokers with normal spirometry. JAMA Intern Med. 2015; 175(9):1539–1549

Schroeder J, McKenzie A, Zach J, et al. Relationships between airflow obstruction and quantitative CT measurements of emphysema, air trapping, and airways in subjects with and without COPD. AJR Am J Roentgenol. 2013; 201:460–470

37 Cystic Lung Disease

Katherine Kaproth-Joslin

37.1 Template

Lungs:
Findings related to pulmonary cysts:
- Zonal distribution: [upper lung predominant/mid-lung predominant/lower lung predominant/diffuse] with [sparing of the costophrenic angles/involvement of the costophrenic angles]. [Free text]
  Location: [primarily paramediastinal/primarily perilymphatic/primarily perivascular/mixed/random]. [Free text]
- Shape: [round/ovoid/irregular/other]; [uniform appearance/variable appearance]; [free text]
- Wall: [thin-walled/thick-walled]; [free text]
- Average size: [ ] mm

Findings not related to pulmonary cysts:
- Nodules: [present/absent]; if present: density: [solid/semisolid/ground-glass]; pattern of distribution: [random/centrilobular/perilymphatic]; zonal distribution: [upper lung predominant/mid-lung predominant/lower lung predominant/diffuse]; size: [ ] mm; [free text]
- Ground-glass opacity: [none/mild/moderate/severe]; [associated with the cysts/not associated with the cysts]; [free-text description/location]
- Interstitial/Septal thickening: [none/mild/moderate/severe]; [free-text description/location]
- Consolidation: [none/mild/moderate/severe]; [free-text description/location]
- Emphysema: [none/mild/moderate/severe]; if present: type [centrilobular/paraseptal/panlobular/mixed]; [free text]
- Other findings: [free text]

Pleura:
- Fluid: [none/small/moderate/large]; [right/left/bilateral]; [simple/complex] [free text]
- Pneumothorax: [none/small/moderate/large]; [right/left/bilateral]; [free text]
- Other: [free text]

Upper abdomen:
- Renal lesions: [present/absent]; if present, density: [solid/macroscopic fat density/simple fluid density/indeterminate]; size: [ ] mm; [free text]
- Other: [free text]

37.2 Stakeholders

Pulmonologists, radiologists, and pathologists.

37.3 Pearls

- A pulmonary cyst is defined as a rounded lucency of the pulmonary parenchyma with a perceptible thin-wall < 3 mm in thickness typically containing air.
- Pulmonary cysts must be distinguished from a cavitary mass, which is typically a gas-filled lesion with a wall thicker than 4 mm and emphysema which does not have a perceptible wall.
- Zonal distribution of the pulmonary cysts in the lungs is one of the most important factors in determining the causative etiology (▶ Table 37.1).
- Attention to cyst size, shape, and presence of any additional findings outside the lung can tailor the differential diagnosis (▶ Table 37.1).
- Lymphangioleiomyomatosis (LAM) is an infiltrative disorder of the smooth muscles characterized by uniform distribution of pulmonary cysts throughout the lung, with involvement of the costophrenic angles (▶ Fig. 37.1). Patients may present with

Table 37.1 Selected causes of cystic lung disease

	Demographics	Zonal distribution	Cyst shape	Wall	Average size Cyst/nodule	Other findings
Lymphangio-leiomyomatosis, sporadic (S-LAM)	Women of childbearing age	Uniform distribution; involves costophrenic angles	Round or oval	Thin walled	Cysts: Typically <1 cm, can be up to 3 cm Nodules: Not typically present	Spontaneous pneumothorax; Chylous effusions; septal thickening may be present
Lymphangio-leiomyomatosis with tuberous sclerosis complex (TCS-LAM)	More common than S-LAM, occurs in 30% of women with TS and 10–15% of men with TS	Uniform distribution; involves costophrenic angles Nodules may also be present: Upper lobe/peripheral	Round or oval	Thin walled	Cysts: Typically <1 cm, can be up to 3 cm Nodules: 1–10 mm	In addition to above, presence of renal angiomyolipomas
Pulmonary Langerhans cell histiocytosis (PLCH)	Young adults 20–40 yo; 90% are cigarette smokers or have smoking exposure	Upper/Mid-lung predominant; sparing of costophrenic angles *Early stage*: Centrilobular/peribronchiolar nodules predominate *Intermediate stage*: Cysts arise secondary to focal dilatation of bronchi and cavitation of nodules *Late stage*: Cysts predominate	Often round but can be bizarre/irregularly shaped	Usually thin walled, can be thick walled	Cysts: Typically <1 cm, can be up to 3 cm Nodules: Typically 1–5 mm, can be up to 1 cm	Pneumothorax; septal thickening may be present
Lymphocytic interstitial pneumonia (LIP)	Mean age 50; female > male; association with other conditions including HIV and connective tissue disease (i.e., Sjogren syndrome)	Diffuse, with mid to lower predominance; typically few in number involving <10% of the lung; often abutting vessels (subpleural or peribronchovascular)	Variable shape, often round or oval; cysts may contain internal structure	Thin walled	Cysts: Typically <1 cm, can be up to 3 cm Nodules: Poorly defined centrilobular nodules, subpleural nodules	*Acute phase*: Ground-glass opacity, consolidation, interlobular septal thickening, thickening of bronchovascular bundles *Chronic phase*: Only cysts may be present
Folliculin gene-associated syndrome (FLCN-S) or Birt-Hogg-Dubé (BHD) syndrome	Autosomal-dominant inheritance; manifest around 30–40 y	Lower lung predominance; paraseptal or paramediastinal involvement common	Variable shape; round, oval, elliptical lentiform, lobulated, or irregular; can septate if large	Thin walled	Cysts: Variable, typically <1 cm, can be up to 8 cm Nodules: not commonly present	Pneumothorax; renal tumors (from oncocytoma to renal cell cancer), may be bilateral and multiple; fibrofolliculomas of skin (face, neck, upper trunk most common); colonic polyposis

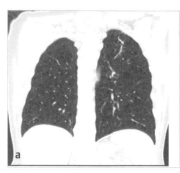
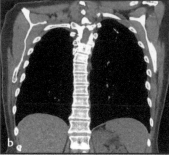

Fig. 37.1 (a, b) Lymphangioleiomyomatosis with tuberous sclerosis complex (TCS-LAM). Coronal computed tomography (CT) images demonstrating uniform distribution of small pulmonary cysts throughout the lungs, including involvement of the costophrenic angles. On mediastinal window, a fat-containing lesion of the left kidney is identified, consistent with an angiomyolipoma.

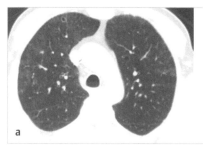
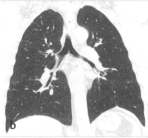

Fig. 37.2 (a, b) Pulmonary Langerhans cell histiocytosis (PLCH). Axial and coronal computed tomography (CT) images demonstrate upper and mid-lung predominant pulmonary cysts and nodules in a patient with an active smoking history. Note that there is sparing of the costophrenic angles.

spontaneous pneumothorax and/or chylous effusions.

- While the spontaneous form of LAM occurs almost exclusively in women childbearing age, the presence of angiomyolipomas in the setting of LAM should raise the suspicion that the patient may have underlying tuberous sclerosis complex, which can occur in both males and females (▶ Fig. 37.1).
- Pulmonary Langerhans cell histiocytosis (PLCH) typically occurs in young adult smokers (95% will have cigarette smoking history) and is characterized by proliferation of Langerhans cells in the bronchiolar and bronchial epithelium, causing the formation of granulomas.
- As PLCH is directly linked to smoke exposure, the pulmonary involvement tends to mimic the typical distribution of emphysema, favoring the upper and mid-lung, with relative sparing of the costophrenic angles (▶ Fig. 37.2).
- PLCH tends to evolve over time, with the early phase characterized by centrilobular and peribronchiolar nodules; the intermediate phase characterized by the development of cysts, in addition to nodules, arising from focal dilatation of the bronchi and the cavitation of the lung nodules; and the late phase predominately characterized by cysts (▶ Fig. 37.2).

- The cysts of PLCH can be bizarre in shape, with the unusual morphology arising when two or more cysts develop in adjacent parenchyma and subsequently fuse to form a distorted cyst.
- Lymphocytic interstitial pneumonia (LIP) is a benign lymphoproliferative disorder characterized by diffuse lymphatic infiltration of the lung, often associated with other conditions such as autoimmune deficiency syndrome and connective tissue diseases, including Sjogren syndrome and systemic lupus erythematosus.
- The cysts found in LIP tend to be few in number, involving less than 10% of the lung, with lower lobe predominance, and are typically found abutting the vessels. Importantly, these cysts occasionally contain internal structures, a finding that is rarely seen in the setting of LAM and PLCH.
- Folliculin gene-associated syndrome (FLCN-S) also known as Birt-Hogg-Dubé (BHD) syndrome is an autosomal-dominant multisystem genetic disorder characterized by cutaneous tumors (fibrofolliculomas), renal tumors (from oncocytoma to renal cell carcinoma), and lower lung predominant cysts (often ovoid/elliptical and paramediastinal or paraseptal in location) (▶ Fig. 37.3).

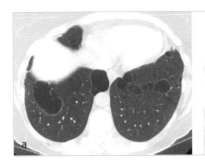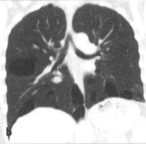

Fig. 37.3 (a, b) Folliculin gene-associated syndrome (FLCN-S) or Birt-Hogg-Dubé (BHD) syndrome. Axial and coronal computed tomography (CT) images demonstrate lower lung predominant cysts with paraseptal and paramediastinal involvement in a patient with known BHD syndrome. Note that many of the cysts are ovoid or elliptical.

Suggested Readings

Beddy P, Babar J, Devaraj A. A practical approach to cystic lung disease on HRCT. Insights Imaging. 2011; 2(1):1–7

Escalon JG, Richards JC, Koelsch T, Downey GP, Lynch DA. Isolated cystic lung disease: an algorithmic approach to distinguishing Birt-Hogg-Dubé Syndrome, lymphangioleiomyomatosis, and lymphocytic interstitial pneumonia. AJR Am J Roentgenol. 2019; 212:1–5

Ferreira Francisco FA, Soares Souza A, Jr, Zanetti G, Marchiori E. Multiple cystic lung disease. Eur Respir Rev. 2015; 24(138):552 564

Gupta N, Vassallo R, Wikenheiser-Brokamp KA, McCormack FX. Diffuse cystic lung disease. Part I. Am J Respir Crit Care Med. 2015; 191(12):1354–1366

Gupta N, Vassallo R, Wikenheiser-Brokamp KA, McCormack FX. Diffuse cystic lung disease. Part II. Am J Respir Crit Care Med. 2015; 192(1):17–29

Raoof S, Bondalapati P, Vydyula R, et al. Cystic lung diseases: algorithmic approach. Chest. 2016; 150(4):945–965

Seaman DM, Meyer CA, Gilman MD, McCormack FX. Diffuse cystic lung disease at high-resolution CT. AJR Am J Roentgenol. 2011; 196(6):1305–1311

38 Lung Cancer Screening

Milena Petranovic and Carol Wu

38.1 Template

Type of scan: [Baseline/3-month follow-up/6-month follow-up/annual/other]
Comparison date(s): [ ]
Prior history of lung cancer (C): [yes/no]
Prior history of malignancy: [yes/no]
Number of nodules: [none/single/multiple < 10 or/multiple > 10]
Dominant nodule: [series number _ image number _]
Lobar location: [right upper lobe/right middle lobe/right lower lobe/left upper lobe/lingula/left lower lobe]
Perifissural: [yes/no]
Endobronchial: [yes/no]
Evolution: [stable/new/enlarging (list prior size)/decreasing (list prior size)/fluctuating]
Attenuation: [solid/subsolid pure ground-glass/subsolid part-solid]
Size: [ ] (mean measurement of long and short axis in millimeters, each measured to one decimal point and mean also rounded to one decimal point [for part-solid nodules both the mean diameter of entire nodule as well as mean diameter of solid component should be recorded])
Margins: [spiculated/smooth/irregular/ill-defined]
Shape: 2D: [round/oval/triangular/lobular, irregular]; 3D: [spherical/flat]
Presence of fat (−50 to −150 HU): [yes/no]
Presence of calcification (> 200 HU): [yes/no]
If yes, type of pattern: [benign (diffuse, central, laminar, popcorn)/nonspecific (punctate, eccentric, amorphous)]
Presence of cavitation: [yes/no]
Incidental findings:
Lungs: [emphysema/infection/interstitial lung disease/other]
Pleura: [effusion/pneumothorax/calcification/mass/other]
Mediastinum and hila: [lymphadenopathy/coronary calcifications moderate or/coronary calcifications severe/cardiomegaly/pericardial effusion/other]
Chest wall and axilla: [soft tissue mass/axillary lymphadenopathy/other]
Bones: [degenerative changes/compression deformity/suspicious lesion/other]
Upper abdomen: [new or enlarging lesion in liver/spleen/pancreas/adrenal/stomach/bowel, lymphadenopathy]
Significant/Actionable incidental finding (S category): [yes/no]
Lung-RADS category:[ ] (Based on Lung-RADS Versions 1.1)
Recommendation for nodule:
[0 Additional lung cancer screening CT images and/or comparison to prior chest CT examination is needed
　　/ 1 LDCT in 12 months
　　/ 2 LDCT in 12 months/return to annual screening on __
　　/ 3 LDCT in 6 months
　　/ 4A LDCT in 3 months/PET-CT/referral to subspecialist or nodule clinic
　　/ 4B LDCT in 3 months/PET-CT/and/or tissue sampling/referral to subspecialist or nodule clinic
　　/ 4X referral to subspecialist or nodule clinic/PET-CT]
Recommendation for incidental finding: _

38.2 Stakeholders

Radiologists, thoracic surgeons, pulmonologists, and primary care physicians.

38.3 Pearls

- Based on the National Lung Screening Trial (NLST) results published in 2011, low-dose chest

CT (LDCT) leads to a 20% reduction in lung cancer mortality compared to chest radiograph. Lung CT Screening Reporting and Data System (Lung-RADS) Version 1.0 established assessment categories and descriptors in 2014, and version 1.1 was released in 2019 (see ▶ Table 38.1).

- Effective dose of radiation of LDCT is estimated to be 1.5 mSv per examination.
- A facility is eligible to receive the ACR Lung Cancer Screening designation if it meets a list of criteria: appropriate equipment and low-dose screening multidetector CT (MDCT) protocol, smoking cessation counseling, trained personnel, and infrastructure for follow-up and reporting. A requirement for structured reporting systems including management recommendations is one of the criteria for designation.
- Comparison with prior imaging studies (and not the previous reports alone) is an important part of nodule evaluation. Comparison should always include the oldest scans available in addition to the most recent prior scan to assess for changes over time, including subtle changes. Growth of a pulmonary nodule by Lung-RADS criteria is defined as an increase in mean diameter of at least 1.5 mm or volume increase of at least 1.8 mm^3.
- Volumetric analysis or volume measurement of nodules may be incorporated into the report in the future to decide on the management of screen-detected nodules. The use of computer-assisted nodule detection and volumetric assessment of nodule size and growth by computer workstation analysis can be valuable adjuncts to the evaluation.
- *Temporary decrease in size* has been reported in lung cancers due to development of fibrosis and/ or atelectasis or resolution of a superimposed

inflammatory change. Therefore, a nodule that decreases in size at short-term follow-up is not necessarily benign.
- Solid nodules with smooth margins, an oval, lentiform or triangular shape, and maximum diameter less than 10 mm or 523.6 mm^3 (perifissural nodules) should be classified as category 2.
- Category 3 and 4A nodules that are unchanged on interval CT should be coded as category 2 and individuals returned to screening (to be performed 12 mo from date of prior baseline or annual scan).
- The *X modifier* is added to nodules that have additional findings that increase suspicion of lung cancer including spiculation (▶ Fig. 38.1), doubling in size of a ground-glass nodule, enlarged lymph nodes, etc.
- Lung-RADS does not address a way to categorize or manage cystic lung lesions. For these lesions, increase in wall thickness or development of a new solid or nodular component should raise concern for malignancy (▶ Fig. 38.2).
- No universally accepted definition of a "significant incidental finding" (S category) exists at the current time though the S designation should be used if further work-up and/or imaging evaluation is required. The definition and the management of a significant

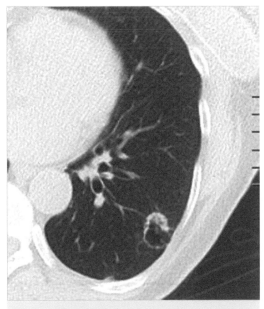

Fig. 38.2 Nodular and/or irregular thickening of a cyst wall is worrisome for primary lung adenocarcinoma.

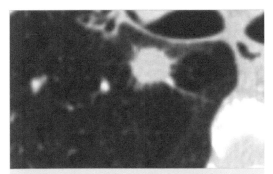

Fig. 38.1 Presence of spiculation such as seen in this nodule is a feature highly concerning for primary lung cancer.

Table 38.1 Lung CT screening reporting and data system

Lung-RADS score/ category descriptor/ risk of malignancy	Screening low-dose chest CT (LDCT) findings[a]	Management
0 Incomplete n/a	• Lungs cannot be evaluated • Prior chest CT comparison exam is being located	Additional lung cancer screening CT images and/or prior chest CT comparison exam needed
1 Negative <1%	• No nodules • Nodules with benign calcifications[a] or fat	Annual LDCT screening in 12 mo
2 Benign appearance or behavior <1%	• Perifissural nodules(s)[b] <10 mm • Solid nodule(s): <6 mm or new <4 mm • Part-solid nodules(s): <6 mm diameter on baseline screening • Nonsolid/ground-glass nodule(s) (▶ Fig. 38.3): <30 mm or ≥30 mm and unchanged or slowly growing • Category 3 or 4 nodules unchanged for ≥3 mo	

3
Probably benign
1–2%
	• Solid nodule(s):
	  ≥6 to <8 mm at baseline or new 4 mm to <6 mm
	• Part-solid nodule(s):
	  ≥6 mm total diameter with solid component <6 mm OR new <6 mm total diameter
	• Nonsolid/ground-glass nodule(s):
	  ≥30 mm on baseline CT or new
		6-mo LDCT

4A
Suspicious
5–15%
	• Solid nodule(s):
	  ≥8 to <15 mm at baseline
	  OR growing <8 mm
	  OR new 6 to <8 mm
	• Part-solid nodule(s):
	  ≥6 mm with solid component ≥6 mm to <8 mm
	  OR with new or growing <4-mm solid component
	• Endobronchial nodule
		3-mo LDCT
		Consider PET-CT if solid component >8 mm

4B Very suspicious >15%	• Solid nodule(s) ≥15 mm OR new or growing, and ≥8 mm • Part-solid nodule(s): Solid component ≥8 mm OR new or growing ≥4-mm solid component	• Chest CT with or without contrast, PET-CT and/or tissue sampling depending on patient comorbidities and probability of malignancy • May recommend 1-mo LDCT for new large nodules developing on annual repeat screening CT that are potentially infectious or inflammatory
4X Very suspicious >15%	Category 3 or 4 nodules with additional features that increase suspicion of malignancy	
S Other	Modifier—may add to category 0–4	As appropriate to the specific finding

Source: Adapted from Lung-RADS Version 1.1 Assessment Categories.
[a]Benign calcification patterns = complete, central, popcorn, concentric rings.
[b]Perifissural nodules with solid with smooth margins, oval, lentiform, or triangular shape and maximum diameter less than 10 mm should be classified as category 2.

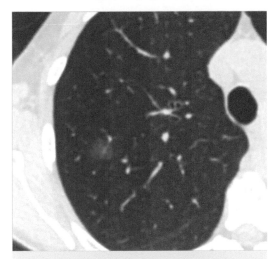

Fig. 38.3 Example of pure ground-glass nodule with preservation of the bronchial and vascular margins and no identifiable solid components.

incidental finding(s) should be decided in conjunction with a multidisciplinary clinical team.

Suggested Readings

ACR Lung CT Screening Reporting and Data System. https://www. acr.org/Clinical-Resources/Reporting-and-Data-Systems/Lung-Rads Accessed June 8, 2019

ACR–STR practice parameter for the performance and reporting of lung cancer screening thoracic computed tomography (CT). https://www.acr.org/-/media/ACR/Files/Practice-Parameters/CT-LungCaScr.pdf

Kazerooni EA, Armstrong MR, Amorosa JK, et al. ACR CT accreditation program and the lung cancer screening program designation. J Am Coll Radiol. 2015; 12(1):38–42

Martin MD, Kanne JP, Broderick LS, Kazerooni EA, Meyer CA. Lung-RADS: pushing the limits. Radiographics. 2017; 37(7):1975–1993

McInnis M, Priyanka J. Explanatory notes: lung cancer screening reporting template. June 2018. https://www.cancercareontario.ca/sites/ccocancercare/files/assets/LungCancerScreeningReporting-TemplateExplanatoryNotes_0.pdf

Munden RF, Carter BW, Chiles C, et al. Managing incidental findings on thoracic CT: mediastinal and cardiovascular findings. A white paper of the ACR incidental findings committee. J Am Coll Radiol. 2018; 15(8):1087–1096

Tsai FR, Chiles C, Carter BW, et al. Incidental findings on lung cancer screening: significance and management. Semin Ultrasound CT MR. 2018; 39(3):273–281

39 Standard Reporting on Chest CT Findings Related to COVID-19

Maya Galperin-Aizenberg, Rachael R. Kirkbride, and Diana Litmanovich

39.1 Template

Findings:
Lung parenchyma:
Ground-glass opacities (GGOs):
- [None]
- [Focal/multifocal]
- [Peripheral/nonperipheral]
- [Basilar predominance/nonbasilar predominance]
- [Rounded morphology/nonrounded morphology]

Consolidation:
[None/isolated lobar or segmental consolidation without GGO/mixed with GGO]
Crazy paving (ground-glass opacities with visible interlobar septal lines): [present/absent]
Reverse halo sign or other findings of organizing pneumonia: [present/absent]
Discrete small nodules (centrilobular, "tree- in-bud"): [present/absent]
Lung cavitation: [present/absent]
Smooth interlobular septal thickening without GGO: [present/absent]
Pleura:
Pneumothorax: [present/absent]
Pleural effusion: [present/absent]
Mediastinum/Vessels:
Evidence of pulmonary embolism: [none/(if present, provide full description)]
Lymph nodes:
Lymphadenopathy: [mild/moderate/extensive] [location]
Impressions:
- [Negative for (COVID-19) pneumonia: No CT findings present to indicate pneumonia./Atypical appearance for (COVID-19) pneumonia: Imaging features are atypical or uncommonly reported for (COVID-19) pneumonia. Alternative diagnoses should be considered./Indeterminate appearance for (COVID-19) pneumonia: Imaging features can be seen with (COVID-19) pneumonia, though are nonspecific and can occur with a variety of infectious and noninfectious processes./Typical appearance for (COVID-19) pneumonia: Commonly reported imaging features of (COVID-19) pneumonia are present. Other processes such as influenza pneumonia and organizing pneumonia, as can be seen with drug toxicity and connective tissue disease, can cause a similar imaging pattern]
- Compared to previous CT, involvement of the lung parenchyma has [increased/decreased/unchanged]

39.2 Stakeholders

Cardiothoracic radiologists, general radiologists, emergency physicians, pulmonologists, primary care physicians, ICU and critical care physicians, oncologists, and cardiologists.

39.3 Pearls

- Coronavirus disease 2019 (COVID-19), caused by severe acute respiratory syndrome coronavirus 2 (SARS-CoV-2), was declared as a pandemic by the World Health Organization (WHO) on March 11, 2020 representing a global international healthcare challenge.
- COVID-19 definitive diagnosis is made by real-time reverse transcriptase-polymerase chain reaction (RT-PCR) assay. While this test was reported to be highly specific, its sensitivity was shown to be variable and not optimal. Test sensitivity in clinical practice may be adversely affected by multiple factors including adequacy

of specimen, specimen type, specimen handling, and stage of infection when the specimen is acquired.

- There is a recognition of the role of chest computed tomography (CT) to inform decisions on whether to test a patient for COVID-19, admit a patient, or provide other treatment, particularly in light of locally constrained resources, such as biochemical testing and availability of personal protective equipment (PPE), although caution should be taken with this approach.
- Most radiology professional organizations and societies in the United States have recommended against performing screening CT for the identification of COVID-19 advising for CT to be used sparingly and reserved for hospitalized, symptomatic patients with specific clinical indications for CT.
- The reported sensitivities and specificities of CT for COVID-19 vary widely likely due to the retrospective nature of the currently published studies, including lack of strict diagnostic criteria for imaging and procedural differences for confirming infection. A recent meta-analysis showed that pooled sensitivity of 94% and the pooled specificity of 37% for the chest CT with positive predictive value ranged from 1.5 to 30.7% and negative predictive value ranged from 95.4 to 99.8%.
- Chest CT findings can precede positivity on RT-PCR. False negative RT-PCR tests have been reported in patients with CT findings of COVID-19 who were eventually tested positive with serial sampling. Alternatively, a normal chest CT

does not exclude COVID-19 infection in appropriate clinical settings.

- The predominant initial imaging pattern on CT is of ground-glass opacification (▶ Fig. 39.1) with occasional consolidation in the peripheries. As the disease progresses, crazy paving consolidation and organizing pneumonia become the dominant CT findings (▶ Fig. 39.2), peaking around 9 to 13 days. Most patients will recover—clearing inside out with the center clearing before the periphery. The worst CT findings peak at about 10 days, by 14 days start to heal, by 26 days the pneumonia is reduced but still present. Symptoms improve before the CT clears. A minority of the patients may progress with extensive multifocal dense consolidations and acute respiratory distress syndrome (▶ Fig. 39.3, ▶ Fig. 39.4, and ▶ Fig. 39.5).
- Pleural effusion, extensive discrete lung nodules, and lymphadenopathy occur in a very small number of cases and suggest bacterial superinfection or another diagnosis.
- When typical features of COVID-19 pneumonia are present in an endemic area as an incidental finding, direct communication with the referring provider to discuss the likelihood of viral infection and to try to reach consensus is recommended.
- When imaging reveals an alternative diagnosis to COVID-19, management is based upon established guidelines or standard clinical practice.
- Descriptive fields in the "Findings" section are optional and should be omitted if the findings are not present.
- For CT examinations that include a portion of the lung, such as CT abdomen, CT neck, CT upper

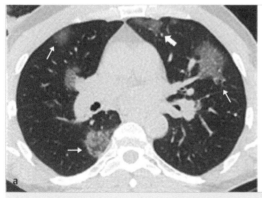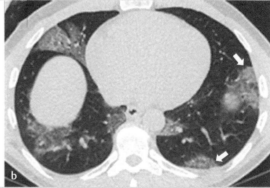

Fig. 39.1 Typical computed tomography (CT) ground-glass opacities (GGO) seen in COVID-19 pneumonia. (a, b) Axial CT images of a 52-year-old male who tested positive for COVID-19 infection shows typical bilateral rounded peripheral GGOs on day 5 post symptoms development (rounded GGO = *thin white arrow*, peripheral GGO = *thick white arrow*).

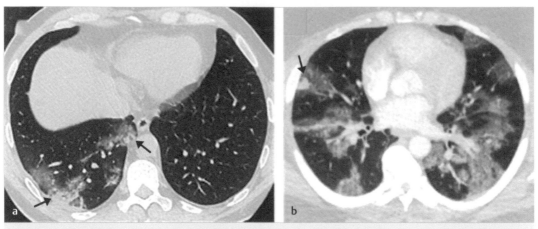

Fig. 39.2 Typical mixed ground-glass and consolidation appearance, and "crazy-paving" appearance in COVID-19 pneumonia. **(a)** Axial computed tomography (CT) in a 40-year-old male who tested positive for COVID-19 infection showing typical mixed ground-glass and consolidative opacities in the right lower lobe (*black arrow*). **(b)** Axial CT in a 40-year-old male who tested positive for COVID-19 infection showing a typical mixed ground-glass and consolidative opacity in the right middle lobe (*black arrow*), and "crazy-paving" appearance in the lower lobes bilaterally.

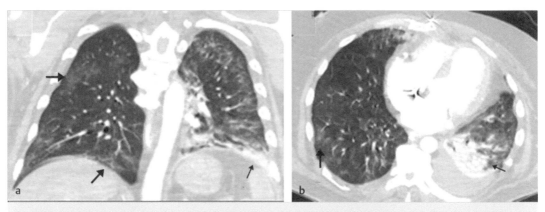

Fig. 39.3 Indeterminate computed tomography (CT) findings for COVID-19. **(a)** Coronary and **(b)** axial contrast-enhanced CT images of a 63-year-old male following coronary artery bypass grafting who has tested positive for COVID-19. The CT images show left basal consolidation with heterogeneous opacification which likely represents atelectasis with the possibility of superimposed infection (*thin black arrows*). Further, scattered bilateral ground-glass opacities (which are resolving compared to prior imaging, not shown) in keeping with resolving acute lung injury (*black arrow*).

extremity, please use the relevant CT template for dictation accepted in your practice for each of the examinations. If the findings in the imaged portion of the lung parenchyma are concerning for COVID-19 pneumonia, please use in the Impression:

"Typical appearance for (COVID-19) pneumonia: Commonly reported imaging features of (COVID-19) pneumonia are present. Other processes such as influenza pneumonia and organizing pneumonia, as can be seen with drug toxicity and connective tissue disease, can cause a similar imaging pattern."

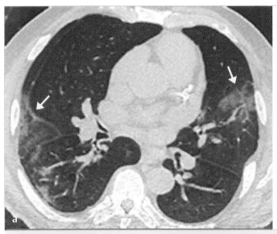
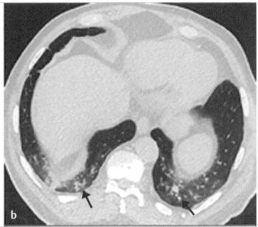

Fig. 39.4 Atypical computed tomography (CT) findings in suspected COVID-19 pneumonia in a 75-year-old with a history of renal transplant who presented with dyspnea. **(a)** Axial CT showing multifocal ground-glass opacities in a pattern suspicious for COVID-19 pneumonia (*white arrows*). **(b)** Axial CT showing bilateral lower lobe bronchiolitis pattern that may be due to a viral or bacterial etiology (*black arrows*).

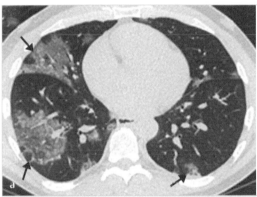
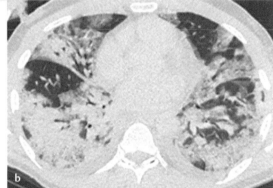

Fig. 39.5 Progression of COVID-19 pneumonia in a 52-year old male who tested positive for COVID-19 pneumonia. **(a)** Axial computed tomography (CT) showing bilateral multifocal ground-glass opacities and consolidation (*black arrows*). **(b)** Axial CT showing progression to bilateral diffuse consolidation with acute respiratory distress syndrome.

Suggested Readings

Ai T, Yang Z, Hou H, Zhan C, Chen C, Lv W, et al. Correlation of chest CT and RT-PCR testing in coronavirus disease 2019 (COVID-19) in China: a report of 1014 cases. Radiology. 2020. doi/10.1148/radiol.2020200642

American College of Radiology. ACR recommendations for the use of chest radiography and computed tomography (CT) for suspected COVID-19 infection. https://www.acr.org/Advocacy-and-Economics/ACR-Position-Statements/Recommendations-for-Chest-Radiography-and-CT-for-Suspected-COVID19-Infection. Updated March 22, 2020. Accessed April 25, 2020

Bai HX, Hsieh B, Xiong Z, et al. Performance of radiologists in differentiating COVID-19 from viral pneumonia on chest CT. Radiology. 2020. doi: 10.1148/radiol.2020200823

Bernheim A, Mei X, Huang M, Yang Y, Fayad ZA, Zhang N, et al. Chest CT findings in Coronavirus Disease-19 (COVID-19): relationship to duration of infection. Radiology. 2020. doi/10.1148/radiol.2020200463

Chung M, Bernheim A, Mei X, et al. CT imaging features of 2019 novel coronavirus (2019-NCoV). Radiology. 2020; 295(1):202–207

Fang Y, Zhang H, Xie J, et al. Sensitivity of chest CT for COVID-19: comparison to RT-PCR. Radiology. 2020. doi: 10.1148/radiol.2020200432

Inui S, Fujikawa A, Jitsu M, et al. Chest CT findings in cases from the Cruise Ship "Diamond Princess" with Coronavirus Disease 2019 (COVID-19). Radiol Cardiothor Imag. 2020; 2(2). doi: 10.1148/ryct.2020200110

Kanne JP, Little BP, Chung JH, Elicker BM, Ketai LH. Essentials for radiologists on COVID-19: an update-Radiology Scientific Expert Panel. Radiology. 2020. doi: 10.1148/radiol.2020200527

Kim H, Hong H, Yoon SH. Diagnostic performance of CT and reverse transcriptase-polymerase chain reaction for coronavirus disease

2019: a meta-analysis. Radiology. 2020. doi: 10.1148/radiol.2020201343

Rubin GD, Ryerson CJ, Haramati LB, et al. The role of chest imaging in patient management during the COVID-19 pandemic: a multinational consensus statement from the Fleischner Society. Chest. 2020; 158(1): 106–116

Salehi S, Abedi A, Balakrishnan S, Gholamrezanezhad A. Coronavirus Disease 2019 (COVID-19): a systematic review of imaging findings in 919 patients. AJR Am J Roentgenol. 2020. doi: 10.2214/ajr.20.23034

Simpson S, Kay FU, Abbara S, et al. Radiological Society of North America Expert Consensus Statement on Reporting Chest CT Findings Related to COVID-19. Endorsed by the Society of Thoracic Radiology, the American College of Radiology, and RSNA. Radiol Cardiothorac Imag. 2020. doi:10.1148/ryct.2020200152

WHO Director-General's opening remarks at the media briefing on COVID-19, March 11, 2020. https://www.who.int/dg/speeches/detail/who-director-general-s-opening-remarks-at-the-media-briefing-on-covid-19. Accessed on April 22, 2020

40 COVID-19 on Chest X-Ray

Maya Galperin-Aizenberg, Rachael R. Kirkbride, and Diana Litmanovich

40.1 Template

> **CXR at presentation:**
> [Multifocal and/or bilateral pneumonia (typical appearance for COVID-19 pneumonia)
> /Focal pneumonia (nonspecific and less typical appearance for COVID-19 pneumonia)
> /Radiographic findings, which are indeterminate for pneumonia (COVID-19 pneumonia or other disease may be present)
> /Negative: No radiographic evidence of pneumonia]
> Current extent of the lung(s) involvement is consistent with [mild/moderate/severe] process
> **Follow-up CXR:**
> [Multifocal and/or bilateral pneumonia (typical appearance for COVID-19 pneumonia)
> /Focal pneumonia (nonspecific and less typical appearance for COVID-19 pneumonia)
> /Radiographic findings, which are indeterminate for pneumonia (COVID-19 pneumonia or other disease may be present)
> /Negative: No radiographic evidence of pneumonia]
> Current extent of the lung(s) involvement is consistent with [mild/moderate/severe] process
> Compared to previous radiograph, Involvement of the lung parenchyma by opacities has [increased/decreased/unchanged]

40.2 Stakeholders

Radiologists, emergency physicians, primary care physicians, pulmonologists, critical care physicians, and ICU physicians

40.3 Pearls

- Chest radiography (CXR) is one of the key tools for pulmonary disease diagnosis and management in the setting of COVID-19 pandemic. See ▶ Table 40.1 for reporting language for CXR findings related to COVID-19.
- Radiographic findings should be considered within the multivariable context of the severity of respiratory disease, pre-test probability, risk factors for disease progression, and critical resource constraints.
- CXR might be insensitive in mild or early COVID-19 infection. However, CXR is often abnormal at the time of presentation when patients experience advanced symptoms in the later stage of the disease (▶ Fig. 40.1).
- **Normal chest radiograph does not exclude COVID-19 infection!**
- CXR can be useful for assessing disease severity and progression, based on zonal assessment of lung involvement.
- CXR can be useful for alternative diagnoses such as lobar pneumonia, suggestive of bacterial superinfection, pneumothorax, and pleural effusion (▶ Fig. 40.2, ▶ Fig. 40.3, and ▶ Fig. 40.4).
- Deploying portable radiography units within an infected patient's isolation room is another factor that may favor CXR, as compared to CT, eliminating the risk of COVID-19 transmission along the transport route to a scanner, particularly in environments lacking personal protective equipment (PPE). The surfaces of these machines can be easily cleaned.
- In stable intubated patients with COVID-19 daily chest radiographs are not adding value and should be avoided to minimize exposure risk of radiology technologists and to conserve PPE.
- Radiographic evidence and severity of pneumonia influences medical triage of patients with suspected COVID-19, by informing decisions on whether to test a patient for COVID-19, admit a patient, or provide other treatment. It should, however, be considered in conjunction with additional factors such as severity of clinical symptoms, prevalence of disease in the local environment, individual risk factors for disease progression, and availability of resources on a system level.

Table 40.1 Reporting language for chest radiography (CXR) findings related to COVID-19

Radiographic classification	CXR findings
Typical appearance	Multifocal bilateral, lower lung predominant
Nonspecific and less typical appearance	Absence of typical findings and Unilateral, central or upper lung predominant distribution
Indeterminate appearance	Pneumonia nonconfidently seen, e.g., bibasilar opacities that could represent pneumonia or atelectasis, or nonspecific interstitial abnormalities
Negative for pneumonia	No lung opacities

Note 1. Findings **atypical** for COVID-19 pneumonia:
- Pneumothorax or pleural effusion
- Pulmonary edema
- Lobar consolidation
- Solitary lung nodule or mass
- Diffuse tiny nodules
- Cavity

Note 2. Reporting language might be used for the following **indications** (but is not limited to):
- Patients with suspected COVID-19 pneumonia
- Assessment or reassessment of patients with COVID-19 pneumonia
- Indications other than suspected viral pneumonia or specifically COVID-19

Note 3. A frontal chest radiograph can be divided into **three zones per lung** (total of six zones):
- Upper zone: apices to the superior portion of the hilum
- Mid zone: between the superior and inferior hilar margins
- Lower zone: between the inferior hilar margins to the costophrenic sulci

Note 4. **Grading** of lung disease on frontal chest radiograph:
- Mild: opacities in one to two lung zones
- Moderate: opacities in three to four lung zones
- Severe: opacities in more than four lung zones

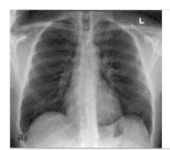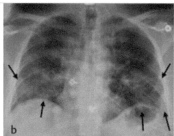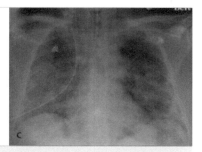

Fig. 40.1 Typical chest radiography (CXR) example of progression from mild to severe COVID-19 pneumonia. A 52-year-old male who tested positive for COVID-19. **(a)** Initial normal CXR performed at diagnosis on the day of the presentation. **(b)** Follow-up CXR a week later shows patchy bilateral multifocal opacities with basilar predominance typical for COVID 19 (*black arrows*). **(c)** Further CXR 6 days later, after the patient deteriorated and was intubated, shows diffuse airspace opacities in keeping with acute respiratory distress syndrome (ARDS).

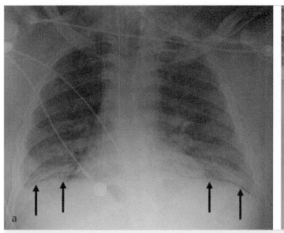

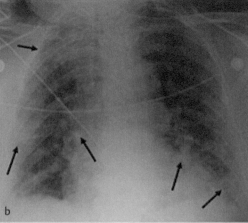

Fig. 40.2 Indeterminate chest radiography (CXR) for COVID-19 pneumonia. **(a)** CXR showing bilateral basal atelectasis (*large black arrows*) and increased pulmonary vascularity in keeping with pulmonary edema. **(b)** CXR in an 87-year-old male showing cardiomegaly, increased pulmonary vascularity, and small pleural effusions in keeping with pulmonary congestion. There are also multifocal bilateral opacities which may represent viral pneumonia (*small black arrows*).

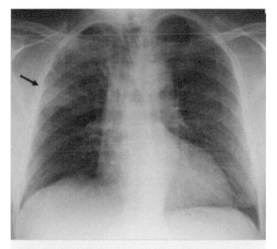

Fig. 40.3 Focal CXR ground-glass opacity. Chest radiography (CXR) of a 61-year-old diagnosed with COVID-19 which shows focal ground-glass opacity (GGO) in the right upper lobe (*black arrow*).

• Recommendations should be discussed and approved with the referring physicians and, ideally, should be center-specific.

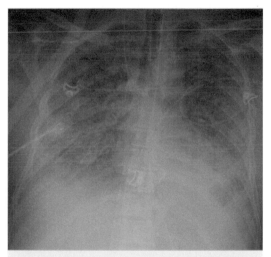

Fig. 40.4 Intubated patient with acute respiratory distress syndrome (ARDS). A 59-year-old male with known asthma and hypertension presented with fever and dyspnea, and tested positive for COVID-19. Chest radiography (CXR) on admission demonstrated consolidation (image not shown). The patient deteriorated and was intubated, and a follow-up CXR 2 weeks later showed severe ARDS (shown) necessitating extracorporeal membrane oxygenation (ECMO) support. The patient later died.

Suggested Readings

Litmanovich DE, Chung M, Kirkbride R, Kicska G, Kanne J. Review of chest radiograph findings of COVID-19 pneumonia and suggested reporting language. J Thorac Imag. 2020. doi: 10.1097/rti.0000000000000541

Rubin GD, Ryerson CJ, Haramati LB, et al. The role of chest imaging in patient management during the COVID-19 pandemic: a multinational consensus statement from the Fleischner Society. Chest. 2020:pii: S0012–3692(20)30673–5. [Epub:ahead of print] PubMed PMID: 32275978; PubMed Central PMCID: PMC7138384

Wong HYF, Lam HYS, Fong AH, et al. Frequency and distribution of chest radiographic findings in COVID-19 positive patients. Radiology. 2019; 201160:201160

Yoon SH, Lee KH, Kim JY, et al. Chest radiographic and CT findings of the 2019 novel coronavirus disease (COVID-19): analysis of nine patients treated in Korea. Korean J Radiol. 2020; 21 (4):494–500

Zhang X, Cai H, Hu J, et al. Epidemiological, clinical characteristics of cases of SARS-CoV-2 infection with abnormal imaging findings. Int J Infect Dis. 2020; 94:81–87–[Internet]

Zhang MQ, Wang XH, Chen YL, et al. Clinical features of 2019 novel coronavirus pneumonia in the early stage from a fever clinic in Beijing. Zhonghua Jie He He Hu Xi Za Zhi. 2020; 43(3):215–218

Section V

Structured Reports in Neuroradiology

Editor: Mark D. Mamlouk

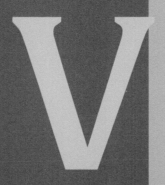

41 Brain Tumors MRI

Brent D. Weinberg and Michael J. Hoch

41.1 Template

Clinical indication:
- Tumor type and mutations: [tumor type] [mutations: IDH +/–, MGMT methylated/unmethylated]
- Surgical history: [none/last surgery date]
- Radiation history: [none/radiation completion date]
- Relevant medications: [none/relevant medications, including bevacizumab (Avastin) or steroids]

Tumor:
- Location: [right/left] [lobe]
- FLAIR: [no change/increasing/decreasing]; [no new sites of FLAIR abnormality/new sites] [optional further description]
- Enhancement: [no change/increasing/decreasing] at primary site; [no new sites of enhancement/new sites] [optional further description]
- Perfusion: [normal/hyperperfusion/hypoperfusion/not performed]
- Diffusion: [abnormal from cellular tumor/normal] [unchanged/new]
- Post-treatment changes: [no unexpected changes/new hemorrhage/new fluid collection]

Other:
- Infarction: [none/new infarct]
- Hemorrhage: [none/new hemorrhage]
- Hydrocephalus: [none/mild/moderate/severe] [unchanged/new]
- Herniation: [none/herniation] [unchanged/new]
- Fluid collection: [none/fluid collection] [unchanged/new]

Impression:
- [Tumor type] status post-treatment. [BT – 0/1a/1b/2/3a/3b/3c/4] (based on scoring from ▶ Table 41.1)
- [Expected post-treatment findings/New unexpected findings]

41.2 Stakeholders

Neurosurgeons, neuro-oncologists, radiation oncologists, and neuroradiologists.

41.3 Pearls

- Magnetic resonance imaging (MRI) reporting in brain tumor patients can benefit from clear and concise reporting that emphasizes the imaging findings used in decision making, including fluid-attenuated inversion recovery (FLAIR), postcontrast enhancement, perfusion, and diffusion.
- The Brain Tumor Reporting and Data System, or BT-RADS, is a structured scoring system devised by a multidisciplinary team which helps categorize MRIs in patients with primary brain tumors.[1]

- BT-RADS was developed as a simplified classification system (scores 0–4) linked to specific management suggestions (▶ Table 41.1).
- Response assessment in neuro-oncology (RANO) criteria[2] was considered in developing BT-RADS, but reporting has been streamlined to maximize ease of use and minimize reliance on ambiguous measurements.
- Compared to conventional free text reports, BT-RADS improved perception of report consistency, decreased ambiguity, and correlation between imaging findings and management decisions.[3]
- Essential history is important. Tumor type and mutations, surgical, medical, and radiation treatment history are included in the report to frame the clinical picture.
- Scoring is based on clinical assessment, timing of therapy and imaging findings seen on FLAIR,

Table 41.1 Post-treatment brain tumor MRI classification according to the BT-RADS scoring system

	Title	Subscore	Imaging description	Management recommendation
0	Not scored		*New baseline*, incomplete study, or otherwise unable to categorize	Continued follow-up, no change
1	Imaging improvement	1a: Improvement	Improvement suspected to reflect *decreasing tumor burden and/or improving treatment effect*	Continued follow-up, no change
		1b: Medication effect	Improvement potentially due to *effect from medications* such as increasing steroids or initiating bevacizumab (Avastin)	Continued follow-up, no change
2	No change		No appreciable change from the prior	Continued follow-up, no change
3	Imaging worsening	3a: Favor treatment effect	Worsening favored to represent *treatment effects*, including radiation therapy and medications	Decreased time interval of follow-up
		3b: Indeterminate	Worsening favored to represent an *indeterminate mix of treatment effect and tumor worsening*	Decreased time interval of follow-up
		3c: Favor tumor progression	Worsening favored to represent *increasing burden of tumor*	Consider change in management vs. Decreased time interval of follow-up
4	Imaging worsening		Worsening *highly suspicious for tumor progression*	Consider change in management

T1-postcontrast, and mass effect. MR perfusion (dynamic susceptibility contrast [DSC] or dynamic contrast-enhanced [DCE]) can be helpful but is not essential to this classification system.

- Imaging findings related to the tumor are reported at the beginning of the report, with nontumor findings at the end.
- The impression of the report includes the tumor type and the overall study score, giving a readily accessible overview.
- New baseline postoperative studies or those with interpretation otherwise confounded (by nondiagnostic images, infection, hemorrhage, lack available priors) are given a SCORE 0.
- Studies with imaging improvement are differentiated into those thought to represent true improvement (SCORE 1A) versus those thought to be improved due to transient medication effects from steroids or bevacizumab (SCORE 1B).
- Patients who show improvement on their first study after starting bevacizumab (Avastin) should be given a SCORE 1B ("pseudoresponse"),

and if improvement is sustained on follow-up it should be given a SCORE 1A for true improvement.

- Clinically stable patients with worsening imaging within the treatment field within 90 days of completing radiation should be given a SCORE 3A, as these findings will often resolve on follow-up imaging ("pseudoprogression") (▶ Fig. 41.1 and ▶ Fig. 41.2).
- Isocitrate dehydrogenase (IDH) and O6-methylguanine-DNA methyltransferase (MGMT) methylated tumors are more likely to have early worsening of imaging after radiation (SCORE 3A) and have a better prognosis.
- Imaging worsening more than 90 days after completing radiation should be viewed with greater suspicion for tumor progression.
- Patients with conflicting imaging findings (such as worsening in only FLAIR or enhancement) should be given a SCORE 3B, as the findings are indeterminate.
- Patients with mild worsening FLAIR and enhancement, mass effect, and clinical worsening more than 90 days after completing

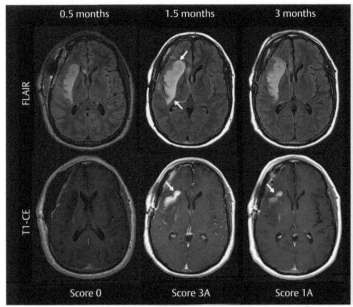

Fig. 41.1 Longitudinal fluid-attenuated inversion recovery (FLAIR) and T1-contrast-enhanced (T1-CE) imaging of a patient with anaplastic astrocytoma treated with surgical debulking and radiation. Initial post-operative imaging was performed 0.5 months after surgical resection to plan radiation therapy and scored as a new baseline, score 0 (column 1). Subsequent follow-up at 1.5 months after surgery demonstrated worsening extent of masslike FLAIR and contrast-enhancing abnormal tissue (column 2, *arrows*), and was given a score 3A. Subsequent follow-up at 3 months showed improvement of immediate radiation-related changes (column 3) and was scored 1A.

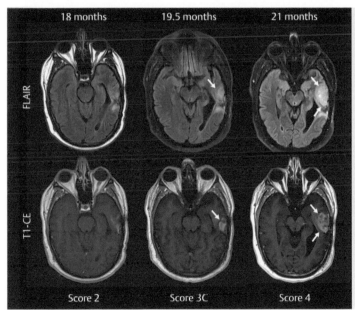

Fig. 41.2 Longitudinal fluid-attenuated inversion recovery (FLAIR) and T1-contrast-enhanced (T1-CE) imaging of a patient with glioblastoma treated with resection and radiation therapy. Routine follow-up imaging 18 months after surgical resection showed stable imaging findings, score 2 (column 1). Subsequent follow-up at 19.5 months after surgery demonstrated worsening abnormal FLAIR and contrast-enhancing tissue (column 2, *arrows*), and was given a score 3C. Subsequent follow-up at 21 months showed progressive worsening of imaging findings (column 3) and was given a score 4.

radiation therapy should be given SCORE 3C, as they are more likely to have tumor worsening.

- Patients with > 25% worsening of the region of abnormal FLAIR or enhancement are highly suspicious for tumor worsening (SCORE 4), consistent with RANO criteria for tumor progression.[2]
- Progressive worsening on more than one follow-up study should be scored as highly suspicious

(SCORE 4). Generally, patients should not have 3C on more than one consecutive study.

- New imaging findings outside the radiation treatment field are more concerning than those within the treated area. New nonenhancing FLAIR lesion outside tumor primary zone is less specific (SCORE 3C) than a new enhancing lesion outside primary treatment zone (SCORE 4).

- For low-grade nonenhancing gliomas, it is essential to compare multiple prior studies (at least 1 year ago if available) to evaluate for slow progression.
- Avoid "pseudoprogression" and "pseudoresponse" in the radiology report as these terms can be confusing to patients and providers. Consider using the terms "treatment effects" and "medication effects," respectively.
- Patients on bevacizumab can have an unchanged enhancing component despite progressing hypercellular tumor seen only as areas of increasing FLAIR and diffusion restriction.
- While the scoring system was devised for primary brain tumors, a similar reporting strategy can be used for central nervous system lymphoma or metastatic disease.

- Additional details on using structured reporting for brain tumors, including detailed criteria for each category, flow charts, and dictation templates, are available at www.btrads.com[4]

References

[1] Weinberg BD, Gore A, Shu HG, et al. Management-based structured reporting of posttreatment glioma response with the brain tumor reporting and data system. J Am Coll Radiol. 2018; 15(5):767–771

[2] Huang RY, Wen PY. Response assessment in neuro-oncology criteria and clinical endpoints. Magn Reson Imaging Clin N Am. 2016; 24(4):705–718

[3] Gore A, Hoch MJ, Shu HG, Olson JJ, Voloschin AD, Weinberg BD. Institutional implementation of a structured reporting system: our experience with the brain tumor reporting and data system. Acad Radiol. 2019; 26(7):974–980

[4] Brain Tumor Reporting and Data System. http://www.btrads.com/. 2018. Accessed March 13, 2019

42 Multiple Sclerosis

Mark D. Mamlouk

42.1 Template

MS Initial Screening
Findings:
Brain parenchyma:
T2 hyperintense white matter lesions:
- **Periventricular:** [no/1–2/3 or more] lesions contacting the ependymal surface
- **Juxtacortical/Cortical:** [none/present]
- **Infratentorial:** [none/present involving the [brainstem/cerebellum/brainstem and cerebellum]]
- **Optic nerve:** [none/present]
- **Cervicomedullary junction:** [none/present]

Enhancing lesions: [<# of enhancing lesions and locations > none]
Reduced diffusion: [none/present (describe)]
Overall disease burden: [none/< 10 lesions/10–20 lesions/> 20 lesions]
Parenchymal atrophy: [none/mild/moderate/severe]
Callosal atrophy: [none/mild/moderate/severe]
Other findings: [none]
Impression:
[Normal MRI brain/multiple white matter lesions that are [typical/atypical/not consistent] with demyelinating disease]
2016 MAGNIMS MRI criteria to establish disease dissemination in space in multiple sclerosis[1]
Involvement of at least two of five areas of the CNS is as follows:
- Three or more periventricular lesions
- One or more infratentorial lesion
- One or more spinal cord lesion
- One or more optic nerve lesion
- One or more cortical or juxtacortical lesion

MS Follow-up
Findings:
Brain parenchyma:
New T2 hyperintense lesions: [<new lesion number and location > none]
Enhancing lesions: [<# of enhancing lesions and locations > none]
Reduced diffusion: [none/present (describe)]
Overall disease burden: [< 10 lesions/10–20 lesions/> 20 lesions]; [no change in multiple [periventricular/periventricular and juxtacortical/periventricular and infratentorial/periventricular, juxtacortical, and infratentorial] white matter lesions compatible with known demyelinating disease]
T1 hypointensities (black holes): [absent/< 5/> 5] and [unchanged/increased] compared to prior exam
Parenchymal atrophy: [none/mild/moderate/severe]
Callosal atrophy: [none/mild/moderate/severe]
Other findings: [none]
Impression:
Demyelinating disease in the [supratentorial/supratentorial and infratentorial] brain, [without/with] active disease and [no change/change] compared to [prior exam date]

42.2 Stakeholders

Neurologists.

42.3 Pearls

- Templates are evidence-based using the magnetic resonance imaging in multiple sclerosis (MAGNIMS) consensus guidelines.[1,2]
- The template is contextual to the pertinent findings related to multiple sclerosis and ensures all relevant points are addressed.[3]
- The screening/diagnostic template guides the interpreter to identify all the necessary lesions to establish a diagnosis of multiple sclerosis (▶ Fig. 42.1). Occasionally, multiple sclerosis can be difficult to diagnose radiologically in the setting of nonspecific white matter lesions.

Because the template follows the MAGNIMS guidelines, the radiologist will be more confident in this diagnosis for the relatively more difficult cases.

- The follow-up template permits rapid reporting because it focuses on the main items required for monitoring disease stability or progression (▶ Fig. 42.2). Many of the fields can be quickly tabbed through, and a final report can often be crafted in a few minutes or less after reviewing the images.
- New lesions in the follow-up template can be annotated with the image number and sequence to make it easy for the referring provider to visualize.
- Comments on the presence or absence of black holes and atrophy are included in the follow-up template to provide information on neuronal loss.[4]

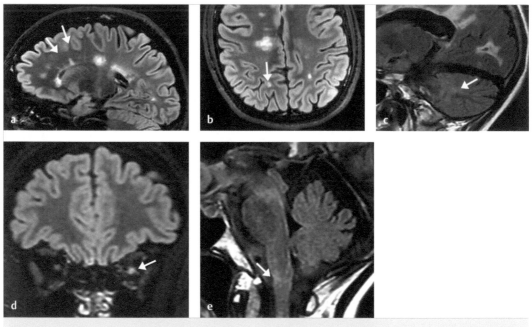

Fig. 42.1 Establishing the diagnosis of multiple sclerosis using the magnetic resonance imaging in multiple sclerosis (MAGNIMS) criteria. Multiple fluid attenuation inversion recovery (FLAIR) images show demyelinating lesions (*arrows*) in the periventricular white matter along the calloseptal interface (**a**), cortical/juxtacortical white mater (**b**), infratentorial white matter (**c**), optic nerve (**d**), and craniocervical junction (**e**).

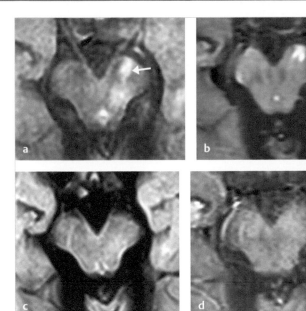

Fig. 42.2 Active demyelination. **(a)** Axial fluid attenuation inversion recovery (FLAIR) and **(b)** axial contrast-enhanced T1-weighted image show a FLAIR hyperintense-enhancing lesion in the left cerebral peduncle (*arrows*). This was not seen on the prior axial FLAIR **(c)** or contrast-enhanced T1-weighted image **(d)**, which is compatible with a new active demyelinating lesion.

References

[1] Filippi M, Rocca MA, Ciccarelli O, et al. MAGNIMS Study Group. MRI criteria for the diagnosis of multiple sclerosis: MAGNIMS consensus guidelines. Lancet Neurol. 2016; 15 (3):292–303

[2] Rovira À, Wattjes MP, Tintoré M, et al. MAGNIMS study group. Evidence-based guidelines: MAGNIMS consensus guidelines on the use of MRI in multiple sclerosis-clinical implementation in the diagnostic process. Nat Rev Neurol. 2015; 11(8):471–482

[3] Mamlouk MD, Chang PC, Saket RR. Contextual radiology reporting: a new approach to neuroradiology structured templates. AJNR Am J Neuroradiol. 2018; 39(8):1406–1414

[4] Sahraian MA, Radue EW, Haller S, Kappos L. Black holes in multiple sclerosis: definition, evolution, and clinical correlations. Acta Neurol Scand. 2010; 122(1):1–8

43 CT/CTA for Acute Stroke Imaging

Anne Catherine Kim

43.1 Template

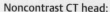

Noncontrast CT head:
Brain parenchyma: [No acute hemorrhage. No mass effect or herniation.] [Gray-white differentiation is maintained.] [White matter is within normal limits for age/nonspecific white matter hypodensities most commonly representing chronic small vessel ischemic changes.]
ASPECTS: [ ]
Ventricles/Extra-axial spaces: [No hydrocephalus or extra-axial fluid collections]
Extracranial structures: [Normal bones and soft tissues. Visualized paranasal sinuses and mastoids are clear.]
CTA head:
[No occlusion or hemodynamically significant stenosis.] [No aneurysm.]
CTA neck:
Great vessels: [Visualized segments are patent.]
Right ICA: [No stenosis or significant plaque.]/[Less than 50% stenosis/Approximately [ ]% stenosis as measured on series [ ], image [ ]/Occluded] by NASCET criteria at the carotid bifurcation with [calcified and soft/calcified/soft] plaque.] [No dissection.]
Left ICA: [No stenosis or significant plaque.]/[Less than 50% stenosis/Approximately [ ]% stenosis as measured on series [ ], image [ ]/Occluded] by NASCET criteria at the carotid bifurcation with [calcified and soft/calcified/soft] plaque.] [No dissection.]
Vertebral arteries: [Patent extracranial segments.] [No dissection.]
Other: [Visualized lung apices are clear. No neck mass or suspicious lymph nodes.] [Bones demonstrate no significant abnormality.]

43.2 Stakeholders

Neurologists, neurointerventionalists, emergency physicians, and others who treat acute stroke.

43.3 Pearls

- Acute stroke is one of the most urgent situations in an emergency department, and imaging is critical to decision-making.
- Stroke imaging has resurfaced as a current hot topic in neuroimaging, as recent large randomized controlled trials demonstrated that acute ischemic stroke can be treated with thrombolytics and/or mechanical thrombectomy (MR CLEAN, ESCAPE, EXTEND IA, SWIFT PRIME, REVASCAT). However, treatment can only be applied within very strict time guidelines.[1] This has led to the common refrain "time is brain."
- Given this time urgency in stroke care, rapid radiology reporting is important. The computed tomography (CT) head and CT angiography (CTA) reports are structured to guide the radiologist and the referring clinician to the key information needed in this emergent situation.
- The CT head structured template focuses on the brain parenchyma, with the first statement indicating the absence or presence of hemorrhage, as this is a contraindication to intravenous thrombolysis.[1]
- The CTA head/neck structured template focuses on five major vessel areas (intracranial, great vessels, right internal carotid artery [ICA], left ICA, and vertebral artery), permitting the radiologist to quickly tab through and report if there is an occlusion or hemodynamically significant stenosis. This is distinct from other CTA reports, which mention each single vessel in the head and neck. The above template will allow the radiologist to report the critical findings in a succinct manner (▶ Fig. 43.1).
- Templated reporting can help provide prompts in this extremely time-compressed situation. For example, an "aneurysm" prompt can remind the radiologist to look for aneurysms, which can potentially complicate mechanical thrombectomy.

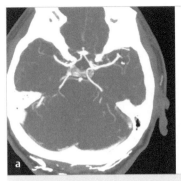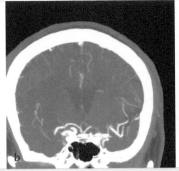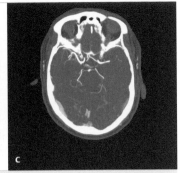

Fig. 43.1 **(a)** Right middle cerebral artery (MCA) M1 occlusion on 10-mm thick slab overlapping axial maximum intensity projections (MIPs). MIPs can greatly aid in the detection of large vessel occlusion, if produced in a timely fashion. **(b)** Occlusion of a right M1 segment of the right MCA in coronal plane MIPs. **(c)** Left MCA occlusion in the M1 segment. Notice also the presence of poor collaterals.

- An "Other" section is included in the CTA template to remind the radiologist to look for incidental findings, such as a pulmonary or neck mass.
- Structured reporting can also include the ASPECTS score,[2] rather than the arbitrary scale of "small/medium/large" when describing ischemia. Patients with poor ASPECTS scores (< 6) were excluded from the late window trial DEFUSE3[3] and may be a factor in which patient is likely or unlikely to benefit from mechanical thrombectomy.
- Magnetic resonance imaging/magnetic resonance angiography (MRI/MRA) is occasionally used for acute stroke imaging but is less accessible.

References

[1] Powers WJ, Rabinstein AA, Ackerson T, et al. American Heart Association Stroke Council. 2018 guidelines for the early management of patients with acute ischemic stroke: a guideline for healthcare professionals from the American Heart Association/American Stroke Association. Stroke. 2018; 49(3):e46–e110

[2] Barber PA, Demchuk AM, Zhang J, Buchan AM. Validity and reliability of a quantitative computed tomography score in predicting outcome of hyperacute stroke before thrombolytic therapy. ASPECTS study group. Alberta Stroke Programme early CT score. Lancet. 2000; 355(9216):1670–1674

[3] Albers GW, Marks MP, Kemp S, et al. DEFUSE3 Investigators. Thrombectomy for stroke at 6 to 16 hours with selection by perfusion imaging. N Engl J Med. 2018; 378(8):708–718

44 Traumatic Brain Injury

Paul M. Parizel and Thijs Vande Vyvere

44.1 Template

Modality: noncontrast CT, contrast CT, CT angiography, MRI

Scalp:

Open scalp wound [location], subgaleal hematoma [location], cephalohematoma [location], foreign bodies [ ]

Skull and craniofacial region:

Skull fracture: calvarium [location], skull base, central and lateral [location], craniofacial [location], pneumo-cephalus [location]

Extra-axial spaces:

Subdural hematoma: [location], [acute, (subacute/chronic)], volumetric assessment (in mL or cc) is the preferred technique (segmentation); if not available, measure size [ ] (width) × [ ] (length) × [ ] (depth) cm/2

Epidural hematoma: [location], probably [arterial/venous], volumetric assessment (in mL or cc) is the preferred technique (segmentation); if not available, measure size [ ] (width) × [ ] (length) × [ ] (depth) cm/2

Subdural hygroma: [location]

CSF spaces:

Intraventricular hemorrhage: [location]

Traumatic subarachnoid hemorrhage: [location: cortical/basal], [degree: trace/moderate/full]

Obstruction hydrocephalus: [degree: mild/moderate/severe]

Cerebral lesions:

Contusion/Intraparenchymal hematoma: [location], volumetric assessment (in mL or cc) is the preferred technique (segmentation); if not available, measure size [ ] (width) × [ ] (length) × [ ] (depth) cm/2

Diffuse or traumatic axonal injury, hemispheres: [location], corpus callosum: [location], thalamus: [location], brain stem: [location]

Cerebral edema: [global]/[location]

Infection: [ ]

Mass effect:

Midline shift, measuring [ ] mm

Herniation: [location]

Cisternal compression: [location], [degree: compressed/obliterated]

Ventricular compression: [location]

Ischemia and blood vessels:

Infarction: [location]

Vessel injury:

- Traumatic dissection: [location]
- Traumatic aneurysm: [location]
- Traumatic occlusion: [location]

Prior/Coexisting pathology:

Old TBI: [location], old stroke: [location], other: [ ]

Cerebral atrophy:

[location] automated volume assessment preferred (segmentation)

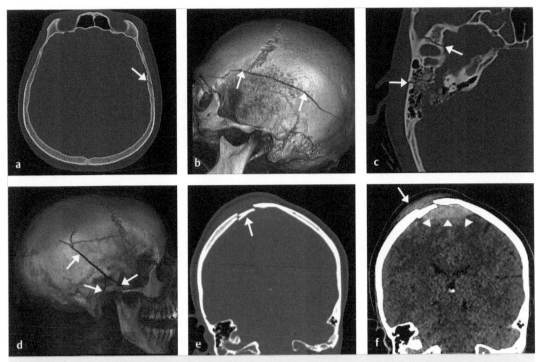

Fig. 44.1 Scalp, skull, and craniofacial structures. **(a, b)** Axial noncontrast computed tomography (NCCT) image and 3D volume-rendering technique (VRT) reconstruction show a linear skull fracture in the calvarium [location: frontoparietal left], *arrows*. **(c, d)** Axial NCCT image and 3D VRT reconstruction show a branched calvarial skull fracture [location: parietotemporal right], extending into the lateral skull base [location: middle fossa, petrous bone right], *arrows*. **(e, f)** Coronal NCCT images. **(e)** Shows a depressed skull fracture [location: parietal right], *arrow*. **(f)** Shows a subgaleal hematoma [location: parietal right], *arrow*, and underlying epidural hematoma [location: parietal right], probably [venous], *arrowheads*.

44.2 Stakeholders

Radiologist, neurosurgeons, neurologists, intensive care physicians, rehabilitation physicians, and psychiatrists.

44.3 Pearls

- In the acute phase after injury, noncontrast computed tomography (NCCT) of the head is the first line of imaging (▶ Fig. 44.1, ▶ Fig. 44.2, ▶ Fig. 44.3, ▶ Fig. 44.4(a, b, c, f), and ▶ Fig. 44.5).[1]
- Whenever there is a discrepancy between the patient's neurological status and the NCCT findings, magnetic resonance imaging (MRI) of the brain should be performed.[1]
- Early-stage MRI, specifically when T2*-gradient echo (GRE) and/or susceptibility weighted imaging (SWI) sequences are included in the protocol, is more sensitive in the detection of

hemorrhagic contusions and axonal injuries (▶ Fig. 44.4d, e).[1]
- There is growing evidence that early-stage MRI can provide important information about patient management, prognosis, and outcome.
- CT- or MR-angiography is being increasingly used in the assessment of traumatic vascular injuries involving the arteries of the skull base and circle of Willis (see ▶ Fig. 44.5d).
- In the subacute to chronic phase after injury, MRI is the preferred technique, especially in traumatic brain injury (TBI) patients with new, persistent, or worsening symptoms. MRI offers a higher sensitivity to detect blood breakdown products (especially hemosiderin) and cerebral atrophy.
- The common data elements (CDEs) have been developed to assist in the interpretation and reporting of TBI lesions, and to standardize data collection.[2]

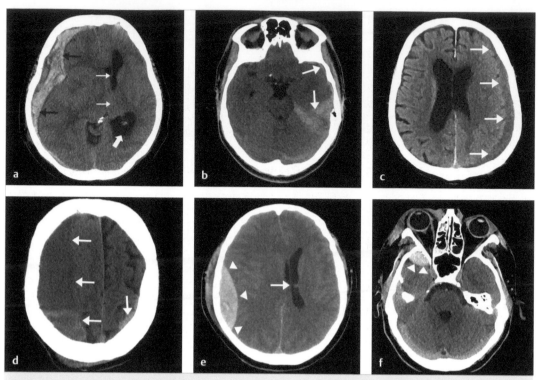

Fig. 44.2 Extra-axial spaces (axial noncontrast computed tomography [NCCT] images). **(a)** Acute subdural hematoma [location: frontotemporoparieto-occipital right], *black arrows* with midline shift, *thin white arrows,* and [severe] obstructive hydrocephalus of the left lateral ventricle, *thick white arrow.* **(b)** Acute subdural hematoma [location: temporal left, tentorial left], *white arrows.* **(c)** Subacute/chronic subdural hematoma [location: frontoparieto-occipital left, frontal right], *white arrows.* **(d)** Acute-on-chronic subdural hematoma [location: frontoparietal right] and acute subdural hematoma [frontoparietal left], *white arrows.* **(e)** Epidural hematoma [location: frontotemporoparietal right], *arrowheads* probably [arterial] with midline shift, *arrow.* **(f)** Epidural hematoma [location: temporal right], probably [venous], *arrowheads.*

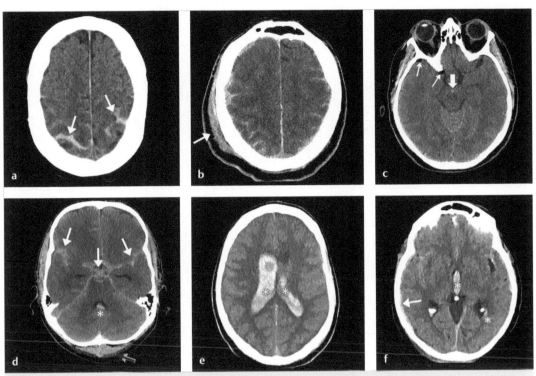

Fig. 44.3 CSF spaces (axial noncontrast computed tomography [NCCT] images). **(a)** Traumatic subarachnoid hemorrhage (tSAH) [location: bilateral cortical], [degree: trace], *arrows*. **(b)** tSAH [location: bilateral cortical], [degree: full] with subgaleal hematoma [location: frontoparietal right]. **(c)** tSAH in the interpeduncular fossa is a common finding [location: basal], [degree: trace], *thick arrow*, in a patient with intracranial air: pneumocephalus [location: temporal right], *thin arrows*. **(d)** Bilateral tSAH [location: basal], [degree: full] [location: cortical], [degree: moderate], *white arrows* and intraventricular hemorrhage (IVH) [location: 4th ventricle], *asterisk*. **(e, f)** Images of the same patient with IVH [location: lateral ventricles, 3rd ventricle], *asterisks*. Notice the subtle subdural hematoma [location: frontotemporal], *arrow*.

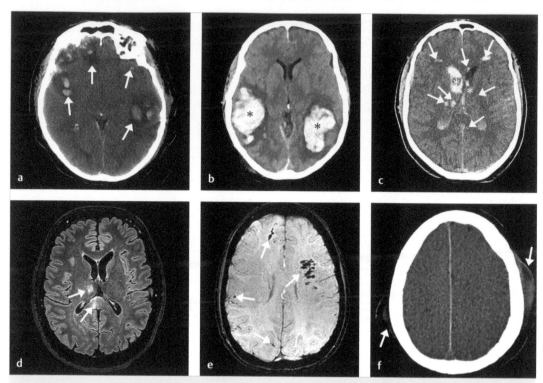

Fig. 44.4 Cerebral lesions (as shown on axial noncontrast computed tomography [NCCT] and magnetic resonance [MR] images). **(a)** Hemorrhagic contusions [location: bilateral frontotemporal], *arrows*. **(b)** Intracerebral hematomas [location: bilateral temporal], *asterisks*. **(c)** Diffuse axonal injuries (DAI), hemispheres [location: bilateral frontal], corpus callosum [location: genu and splenium left], thalamus: [location: right], *arrows* and intraventricular hemorrhage (IVH) [location: lateral ventricles], *asterisks*. **(d)** Traumatic axonal injury (TAI), shown on an axial fluid attenuation inversion recovery (FLAIR) image with spectral fat saturation, in the corpus callosum [location: splenium right] and thalamus [location: right], *arrows*. **(e)** DAI, shown on an axial susceptibility weighted imaging (SWI) image; in the hemispheres [location: bilateral frontal, occipital right], *arrows*. **(f)** Cerebral edema [global]. Notice the loss of gray-white matter differentiation and pronounced cortical sulcal effacement and bilateral subgaleal hematomas [location: parietal right and frontoparietal left], *arrows*.

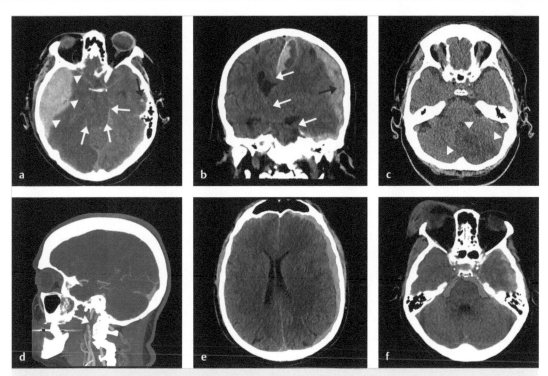

Fig. 44.5 Mass effect, posttraumatic ischemia, blood vessel injuries, and volumetric assessment. (a) Epidural hematoma [location: parietotemporal right], *arrowheads*, causing cisternal compression [location: suprasellar, ambient, quadrigeminal cistern], [degree: obliterated], *white arrows*. Notice the presence of a contralateral contusion [location: temporal left], *black arrow*. (b) Subdural hematoma [location: frontotemporoparieto-occipital left] causing transtentorial brain herniation, *white arrows* [location: subfalcine, central and uncal left]. (c) Cerebellar infarction [location: cerebellum left, posterior inferior cerebellar artery], *arrowheads*. (d) Vascular dissection [location: internal carotid artery right], *arrow*. (e) Example of volumetric assessment of subdural hematoma [location: frontotemporoparieto-occipital left]. (f) Example of volumetric assessment of the basal cisterns [location: ambient and prepontine cistern].

Table 44.1 Rotterdam CT scoring system[4]

Basal cisterns	
Normal	0 points
Compressed	1 point
Absent	2 points
Midline shift	
No shift or 5 mm	0 points
Shift > 5 mm	1 point
Epidural mass lesion	
Present	0 points
Absent	1 point
IVH or tSAH	
Absent	0 points
Present	1 point
Sum score	**+1 point**

Abbreviations: IVH, intraventricular hemorrhage; tSAH, traumatic subarachnoid hemorrhage.
Source: Adapted from Maas AI et al 2005.[4]

- Research shows that structured (synoptic) reporting templates increase interpretation accuracy and reduce the number of missed critical diagnoses.[3]
- Quantitative measurements provide essential information to guide patient management, e.g., surgical vs. nonsurgical treatment. Examples include lesion volume assessment (in cc/mL) and measurement of midline shift (in mm).
- There are multiple CT grading systems in existence which take into account specific qualitative features to predict mortality and unfavorable outcomes (e.g., the Marshall CT classification, the Rotterdam CT score [▶ Table 44.1],[4] Helsinki CT score, etc.). The NeuroImaging Radiological Interpretation System (NIRIS) is a newly developed and promising scoring system that suggests actions for patient management, in addition to predicting mortality (▶ Table 44.2).[5]
- The incorporation of quantitative NCCT features (i.e., lesion volume, basal cistern volume, and midline shift) significantly improves outcome prediction, when compared to qualitative NCCT features only (see ▶ Fig. 44.4e, f).[6]

Table 44.2 Neuroimaging radiological interpretation system (NIRIS)

Category	Definition	Patient management/actions
NIRIS 0	No abnormal finding	Discharge from the ED
NIRIS 1	Fracture ±	Follow-up neuroimaging and/or admit for observation
	Extra-axial hematoma, intraparenchymal hematoma/contusion < 0.5 mL ±	
	Subarachnoid hemorrhage	
NIRIS 2	Extra-axial hematoma, intraparenchymal hematoma/contusion > 0.5 mL ±	Admit to a more advanced care unit
	Diffuse axonal injury ±	
	Intraventricular hemorrhage ±	
	Mild hydrocephalus ±	
	Midline shift 0–5 mm	
NIRIS 3	Extra-axial hematoma, intraparenchymal hematoma/contusion > 5 mL ±	Consider neurosurgical procedure (ventricular drain, burr hole, craniotomy/craniectomy, surgical drainage/evacuation of hematoma)
	Moderate hydrocephalus ±	
	Midline shift > 5 mm ±	
	Focal herniation	
NIRIS 4	Extra-axial hematoma, intraparenchymal hematoma/contusion > 25 mL ±	High risk of TBI-related death
	Severe hydrocephalus ±	
	Diffuse herniation/duret hemorrhage	

Abbreviations: ED, emergency department; TBI, traumatic brain injury.
Source: Adapted from Wintermark M, Li Y, Ding VY, et al.[5]

- The template presented in this chapter allows computation of all currently validated CT and MRI-grading scales.

References

[1] Parizel PM, Van Goethem JW, Özsarlak O, Maes M, Phillips CD. New developments in the neuroradiological diagnosis of craniocerebral trauma. Eur Radiol. 2005; 15(3):569–581

[2] Haacke EM, Duhaime AC, Gean AD, et al. Common data elements in radiologic imaging of traumatic brain injury. J Magn Reson Imaging. 2010; 32(3):516–543

[3] Evans LR, Fitzgerald MC, Varma D, Mitra B. A novel approach to improving the interpretation of CT brain in trauma. Injury. 2018; 49(1):56–61

[4] Maas AI, Hukkelhoven CW, Marshall LF, Steyerberg EW. Prediction of outcome in traumatic brain injury with computed tomographic characteristics: a comparison between the computed tomographic classification and combinations of computed tomographic predictors. Neurosurgery. 2005; 57(6):1173–1182, discussion 1173–1182

[5] Wintermark M, Li Y, Ding VY, et al. Neuroimaging radiological interpretation system for acute traumatic brain injury. J Neurotrauma. 2018; 35(22):2665–2672

[6] Yuh EL, Cooper SR, Ferguson AR, Manley GT. Quantitative CT improves outcome prediction in acute traumatic brain injury. J Neurotrauma. 2012; 29(5):735–746

45 NI-RADS (Neck Imaging Reporting and Data System)

Xin (Cynthia) Wu and Ashley Hawk Aiken

45.1 Template

Exam: CT neck soft tissue with contrast
Clinical indication:
Subsite:
HPV status:
Surgery date: [N/A]
Chemoradiation completion date: [N/A]
Technique: Helical CT examination of the neck with IV contrast. Sagittal and coronal reformations were generated. If applicable, point-of-care testing was approved following departmental protocol
Comparison: [none]
Findings:

- Post-surgical changes: [none]
- Primary site: [no evidence of recurrent disease]
- Neck: [no pathologically enlarged, necrotic, or otherwise abnormal lymph nodes]
- Post-treatment changes: [expected including supraglottic mucosal edema and thickening of the skin and subcutaneous soft tissues]
- Aerodigestive tract: [no findings to suggest a second primary]
- Brain, orbits, spine, and lungs: [no aggressive lesions suspicious for metastatic involvement]

Impression:
Primary: [1, expected post-treatment changes in the neck without evidence of recurrent disease in the primary site]
Neck: [1, no abnormal lymph nodes]
NI-RADS numerical suspicion legend:
NI-RADS is a standardized reporting system for follow-up of treated head and neck cancers
Primary
0: New baseline study: need priors to assign final score
1: No evidence of recurrence: routine surveillance
2: Low suspicion
a) Superficial abnormality (skin, mucosal surface): direct visual inspection
b) Ill-defined deep abnormality: short interval follow-up* or PET

3: High suspicion (new or enlarging discrete nodule/mass): biopsy if clinically indicated
4: Definitive recurrence (path proven or clinical progression)
Neck
0: New baseline study: need priors to assign final score
1: No evidence of recurrence: routine surveillance
2: Low suspicion (ill-defined): short interval follow-up or PET
3: High suspicion (new or enlarging lymph node): biopsy if clinically needed
4: Definitive recurrence (path proven or clinical progression)
*Short interval follow-up: 3 months at our institution

45.2 Stakeholders

Head and neck surgeons, radiation oncologists, and medical oncologists.

45.3 Pearls

- NI-RADS was developed for contrast-enhanced computed tomography (CECT) surveillance imaging with or without positron emission tomography (PET) in patients with treated head-and-neck cancer, in accordance with ACR's charge to deliver patient-centered, data-driven, outcomes-based care.[1,2]

- The NI-RADS scoring system can be adapted for magnetic resonance imaging (MRI) head and neck cancer surveillance.
- NI-RADS provides numerical levels of suspicion to guide patient care, with standardized linked management recommendations. It also generates data-mineable reports to further optimize surveillance algorithms, accuracy, interobserver variability, and highlight radiologists' added value in patient care.
- Five numerical categories are used for primary site as well as regional nodal metastatic disease in the neck, each of which is tied to a specific management recommendation. If the NI-RADS template is used for interpretation of whole-body PET-CT imaging, an "M" score can be added for evaluation of distant/systemic metastatic disease.
- Initial surveillance at our institution is CECT with concurrent PET, 12 weeks after completing head-and-neck cancer treatment.
- Initial data on performance of NI-RADS in a cohort of both CECT and PET/CECT surveillance at different times shows significant discrimination between the NI-RADS groups,

with NI-RADS-1 recurrence rate of 3.5%, NI-RADS-2 recurrence rate of 17%, and NI-RADS-3 recurrence rate of 59.4%.[3]

- NI-RADS-0 should only be assigned if there are known prior examinations which could be obtained for comparison. Otherwise, a best attempt should be made at assigning a NI-RADS category of 1–3 (▶ Fig. 45.1, ▶ Fig. 45.2, and ▶ Fig. 45.3).
- NI-RADS-2 category is further divided into 2a and 2b categories, depending on whether the low-suspicion abnormality is superficial (and thus amenable to direct or endoscopic inspection ▶ Fig. 45.4) or deep (and thus necessitating follow-up with imaging). NI-RADS category 2 should be considered when CECT and PET findings are discordant.
- An established NI-RADS lexicon can be used in the dictation fields for primary and nodal disease, each of which corresponds to a NI-RADS category (▶ Table 45.1).
- At our institution, the legend for NI-RADS categories and corresponding recommendations are incorporated to the bottom of every standardized head-and-neck cancer follow-up report to facilitate clear communication between radiologists, our referrers, and our patients. It is important to clearly label and distinguish the legend from the impression.

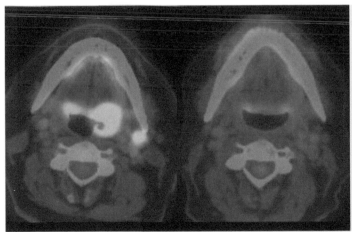

Fig. 45.1 Primary Neck Imaging Reporting and Data System (NI-RADS-1): 70-year-old male patient with T4N2bM0 P16 + squamous cell carcinoma (SCCA) of the left tonsil, with pretreatment fused positron emission tomography-computed tomography (PET-CT) demonstrating fluoro-deoxy-glucose (FDG) avidity in the left tonsillar fossa and a pathologic left level IIA lymph node (left). Three months after treatment with chemoradiation, the fused PET-CT image shows no evidence of residual abnormal soft tissue, enhancement, or FDG uptake within the tonsillar fossa or tongue base (right).

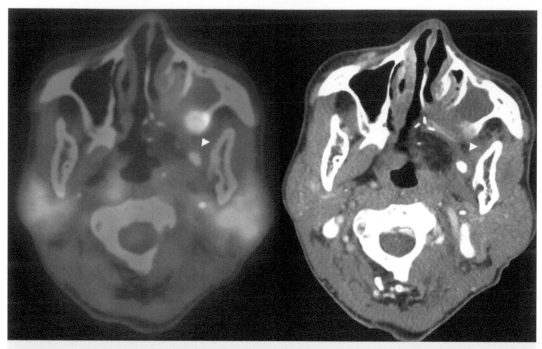

Fig. 45.2 Primary Neck Imaging Reporting and Data System (NI-RADS-3): 61-year-old female patient with large left palate polymorphous low-grade adenocarcinoma, status post maxillectomy and radial free flap reconstruction and pharyngoplasty, with surgical pathology suspicious for positive resection margins. Patient decline chemoradiation. A 4-month follow-up examination demonstrated focal nodular-enhancing soft tissue with osseous erosion along the left posterior maxillary wall resection margin, with corresponding fluoro-deoxyglucose (FDG) uptake (arrowheads), highly suspicious for recurrent/residual disease.

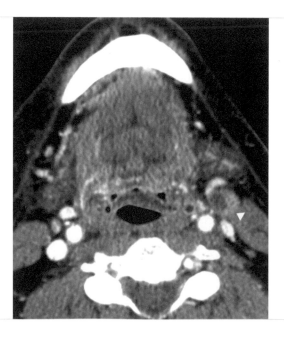

Fig. 45.3 Neck Imaging Reporting and Data System (NI-RADS-3): 59-year-old male patient who was treated for a thyroglossal duct remnant squamous cell carcinoma (SCCA) with wide local excision, central neck dissection, and concurrent adjuvant chemoradiation. Three months after conclusion of treatment, contrast-enhanced computed tomography (CECT) shows a new centrally necrotic, round left level IIA lymph node not present on pre-treatment imaging (arrowhead).

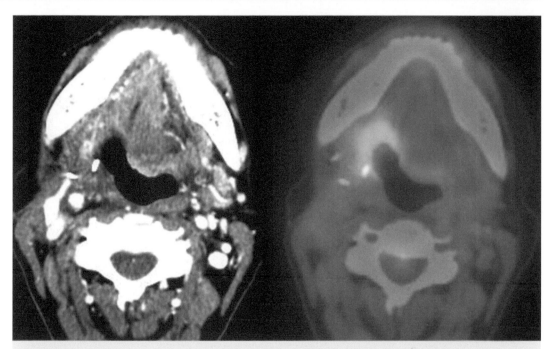

Fig. 45.4 Primary Neck Imaging Reporting and Data System (NI-RADS-2a): 56-year-old female with right base of tongue high-grade mucoepidermoid carcinoma. Three months after treatment with transoral robotic surgery and chemoradiation, contrast-enhanced computed tomography (CECT) shows ulceration at the right tongue base with minimal deep enhancement and no nodular or masslike enhancement. The fused positron emission tomography-computed tomography (PET/CT) image shows intense mucosal fluoro-deoxyglucose (FDG) uptake at the primary site. Given that this abnormality is mucosal, and the relative discordance between CECT and PET (PET much more suspicious than CECT), this should be assigned a "2a." Direct inspection of this site demonstrated radiation mucositis.

Table 45.1 NI-RADS lexicon, corresponding categories, and recommendations

Primary			Nodal		
Lexicon	NI-RADS category	Recommendation	Lexicon	NI-RADS category	Recommendation
Non-mass-like soft tissue, or hypoenhancing distortion of soft tissue and fat planes	1	Routine surveillance	Residual nodal tissue with no FDG uptake relative to background	1	Routine surveillance
Mucoid density, or diffuse linear enhancement indicating benign radiation mucositis	1	Routine surveillance	Residual nodal tissue with mild FDG uptake relative to background	2	Short interval follow-up or PET
Focal mucosal enhancement or FDG uptake	2a	Direct visual inspection	Growing nodal tissue along expected nodal drainage without definite abnormal morphology	2	Short interval follow-up or PET
Ill-defined, mildly enhancing deep masses, possibly with mild FDG uptake	2b	Short interval follow-up or PET	Residual nodal tissue with intense FDG uptake relative to background	3	Biopsy if clinically needed
Discrete, robustly enhancing masses, possibly with intense FDG uptake	3	Biopsy if clinically indicated	Growing nodal tissue with abnormal morphology or intense FDG uptake	3 or 4	Biopsy if clinically needed

Abbreviations: FDG, fluoro-deoxyglucose; NI-RADS, Neck Imaging Reporting and Data System; PET, positron emission tomography.
Source: Adapted from Aiken AH, Rath TJ, Anzai Y, et al 2018.[2]

References

[1] Aiken AH, Farley A, Baugnon KL, et al. Implementation of a novel surveillance template for head and neck cancer: neck imaging reporting and data system (NI-RADS). J Am Coll Radiol. 2016; 13(6):743–746.e1

[2] Aiken AH, Rath TJ, Anzai Y, et al. ACR neck imaging reporting and data systems (NI-RADS): a white paper of the ACR NI-RADS Committee. J Am Coll Radiol. 2018; 15(8):1097–1108

[3] Krieger DA, Hudgins PA, Nayak GK, et al. Initial performance of NI-RADS to predict residual or recurrent head and neck squamous cell carcinoma. AJNR Am J Neuroradiol. 2017; 38 (6):1193–1199

46 Dementia

Mark D. Mamlouk

46.1 Template

Findings:
Brain volume: [no age-significant/mild/moderate/severe] atrophy] [<location > global without lobar predilection or asymmetry./Regional atrophy, [describe]]
Hippocampal volume: [normal/mildly/moderately reduced/severely reduced]
Brainstem/Cerebellum: [normal volume and signal intensity; no imaging findings of progressive supranuclear palsy, multiple system atrophy, or other primary cerebellar neurodegenerative condition]
Cortex/Basal ganglia: [no evidence of prior insult, abnormal mineralization, prion disease, or autoimmune encephalitis]
Ischemia:
Infarction: [<infarct, attention angular gyrus, thalamus, basal forebrain, PCA territory, ACA territory > none]
Chronic small vessel disease: [<attention to the deep component > absent/mild/moderate/severe]
Cerebral microhemorrhages: [<attention location and pattern > none]
Mass: [none]
Ventricles: [no hydrocephalus/ex-vacuo dilatation/hydrocephalus, [describe]]
Extra-axial fluid collections: [none]
Other findings: [none]
Impression:
[No MRI evidence of a neurodegenerative process]

46.2 Stakeholders

Neurologists, psychiatrists, and general practitioners.

46.3 Pearls

- This template guides the reader to report on the most common causes of dementia. It is arranged in a checklist fashion to ensure all pertinent points are addressed.[1]
- A discussion of brain volume is the first item discussed to direct the radiologist and referring provider to this important point (▶ Fig. 46.1). The degree of hippocampal volume loss is described as none/mild/moderate/severe; however, if the radiologist prefers, he/she can also use the medial temporal lobe atrophy score.[2]
- The brainstem and cerebellum are mentioned, which can be overlooked on imaging due to their uncommon pathologies, e.g., multiple system atrophy (▶ Fig. 46.2).
- Causes of rapidly progressive dementia are addressed, including prion disease (▶ Fig. 46.3) and autoimmune encephalitis.

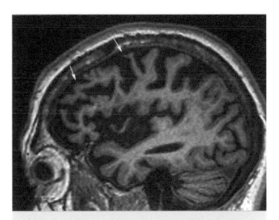

Fig. 46.1 Sagittal spoiled gradient recalled echo shows severe volume loss of the frontal and superior temporal lobes with a knifelike appearance (*arrows*), which is compatible with frontotemporal dementia.

- The template reminds the radiologist to identify infarcts in unique locations that can result in dementia.
- Other common entities such as amyloid angiopathy (▶ Fig. 46.4) and normal pressure hydrocephalus (▶ Fig. 46.5) are included.

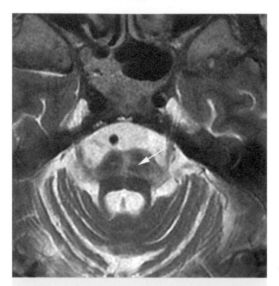

Fig. 46.2 Axial T2-weighted image shows volume loss of the medulla with hyperintense signal in a cruciform appearance (*arrow*)—the classic "hot cross buns" of multiple system atrophy, cerebellar type.

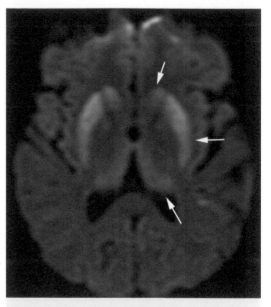

Fig. 46.3 Axial diffusion-weighted imaging shows symmetric hyperintense signal (*arrows*) in the caudate nuclei, putamina, and dorsomedial thalami, consistent with prion disease.

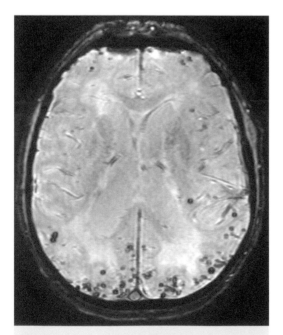

Fig. 46.4 Axial susceptibility-weighted imaging shows several microhemorrhages throughout the brain but predominantly in a lobar distribution, which is in keeping with cerebral amyloid angiopathy.

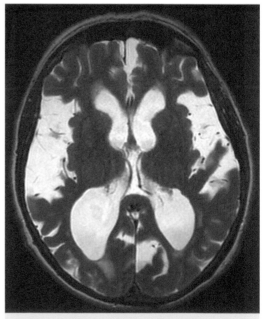

Fig. 46.5 Axial T2-weighted imaging shows enlargement of the lateral ventricles and Sylvian fissures that is disproportionate to the remaining sulci, compatible with normal pressure hydrocephalus.

References

[1] Mamlouk MD, Chang PC, Saket RR. Contextual radiology reporting: a new approach to neuroradiology structured templates. AJNR Am J Neuroradiol. 2018; 39(8):1406–1414

[2] Duara R, Loewenstein DA, Potter E, et al. Medial temporal lobe atrophy on MRI scans and the diagnosis of Alzheimer disease. Neurology. 2008; 71(24):1986–1992

Section VI

Structured Reports in Cardiovascular Imaging

Editors: Rodrigo Salgado and Diana Litmanovich

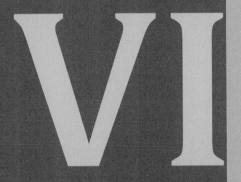

VI

47 Coronary CT-Angiography (CTA)

Rodrigo Salgado

47.1 Template

Clinical history:
Relevant clinical history and previous examinations include: [provide additional information]
Medication profile:
The following medication was administered before the administration:
- Nitroglycerine [sublingual/spray]: [yes/no] with a dose of ___ (if applicable)
- Intravenous β-blocker: [yes/no] with a dose of ___ mL (if applicable)
- Other medication: (provide additional information if applicable)

CT acquisition:
Intravenous contrast medium [was used/was not used/was contraindicated]
[Prospective/retrospective] ECG-triggering was used, with an average heart rate of ___ BPM
Image quality was [excellent/good/moderate/poor]
Cardiac and valvular morphology:
The cuspidity of the aortic valve is [tricuspid/bicuspid/non-assessable]
There [is/is no] [thickening/calcification] of the aortic and mitral valve annulus
There is [no/presence of] left ventricular hypertrophy. This hypertrophy is [concentric/apical/septal/asymmetric] with a maximum thickness of [ ] mm (when applicable)
There is [no/presence] of intracardiac thrombus. [Provide additional details when present]
There are [no/present] signs of an old myocardial infarction. [Provide additional details when present]
Pericardium thickness is [normal/increased] with [presence/absence] of pericardial [effusion/calcification]
Coronary calcifications:
Coronary calcification quantification was performed with following results:

	LM	LAD	RCA	LCX	Total
Agatston-score					
Calcium mass (mg)					
Calcium volume (mm³)					

The total Agatston-score corresponds with the __ % percentile based on age and gender.
Coronary anatomy:
Coronary dominance: [left/right/left-codominant]
Coronary anatomic anomalies are [absent/present]. [Provide additional details when present]

Coronary artery segment	Normal/abnormal	Vessel size and length	Plaque morphology	Stenosis severity
LM				
LAD (proximal/mid/distal)				
D1				
D2				
LCX (proximal/distal)				

Coronary artery segment	Normal/abnormal	Vessel size and length	Plaque morphology	Stenosis severity
OM1				
OM2				
RCA (proximal/mid/distal)				
PDA (right/left)[a]				
PLB (right/left)[a]				

[a]Choice depending on coronary dominance.

Guidelines for interpretation are given in ▶ Table 47.1.

The lesion with the highest-grade stenosis is located in [specify location] with a stenosis of [specify grading].

Noncardiac findings:

There [are/are not] additional nonvascular findings which may influence the immediate and short-term outcome. (Mention these findings when present)

There [are/are not] additional nonvascular findings which may influence the mid- and long-term short outcome. (Mention these findings when present)

Conclusion:

Based on our findings, the following recommendation is made:

(Choose between following options)

- Reassurance. Consider noncoronary causes of chest pain
- Nonobstructive coronary artery disease. Findings to be integrated with other results for optimization of therapy
- Obstructive coronary artery disease. Further investigation is warranted
- Inconclusive examination for obstructive coronary artery disease

Optional:

CAD-RADS score: [0–5/N]

Table 47.1 Recommendations for reporting coronary CTA examinations

Vessel size and length	
Choose between [small/large] and [short/long] vessel segment	
Plaque morphology	
Choose between calcified/noncalcified/mixed plaque Optional: add information on plaque surface delineation (smooth/irregular) and presence of positive remodeling	
Grading scale for stenosis severity	
0%	No visible stenosis
1–24%	Minimal stenosis
25–49%	Mild stenosis
50–69%	Moderate stenosis
70–99%	Severe stenosis
100%	Occluded

Abbreviation: CTA, computed tomography angiography.

47.2 Stakeholders

General and cardiovascular radiologists, as well as cardiologist involved in work-up of a patient with nonspecific chest pain.

47.3 Pearls

- The technical quality of a coronary CTA examination is paramount to achieve diagnostic results.[1] A low and stable heart rate therefore remains, even with todays' high-end systems, an important requisite to achieve high image quality at the lowest possible radiation exposure.
- Medication is in this respect administered to achieve two goals: to lower the heart rate (usually to < 65 BPM if possible) and to achieve better dilatation of the coronary arteries. β-Blockers and nitroglycerine (either sublingually or through a spray) are therefore respectively used. Contraindications must be observed.[2]
- Quantification of coronary calcium calculated using the Agatston-method has emerged as a powerful prognostic factor, delivering long-term

risk stratification information beyond traditional risk factors.[3] This examination must be performed under the known standardized conditions (e.g., 120 kV). Dose-reduction techniques like the use of iterative reconstruction methods and lower kV values are not recommended, as they may influence the calculated value. Furthermore, Agatston-score values tend to slightly differ across different manufacturers for the same patient. Comparison of results not performed on the same system should therefore be made with caution.
- One of the most important tasks of a coronary CTA examination is to exclude significant coronary artery disease (▶ Fig. 47.1). Therefore, when in doubt regarding the degree of stenosis, it is safer to recommend further examination than to assume nonobstructive disease. Stenosis evaluation may be especially difficult in the presence of extensive coronary artery calcifications (▶ Fig. 47.2).
- CT-derived fractional flow reserve (FFR) measurements are increasingly being validated as a powerful method to determine the hemodynamic significance of intermediate coronary stenoses, a value < 0.80 indicating a hemodynamic significant lesion. When available, these results must be integrated in the report.
- Various societies have issued guidelines and other documents regarding the use and reporting of coronary CTA examinations.[4] A recent standardized reporting system promotes the use of a CAD-RADS score to facilitate

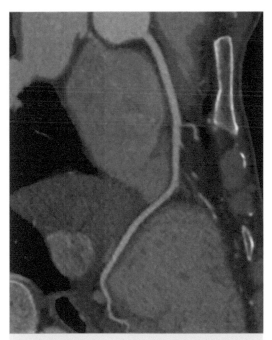

Fig. 47.1 Completely normal left anterior descending (LAD) coronary artery. Coronary computed tomography angiography (CTA) has a very high negative predictive value for significant coronary artery disease, and can therefore avoid an invasive angiography in cases of chest pain of undetermined origin.

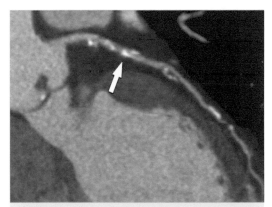

Fig. 47.2 Extensive calcification in the proximal left anterior descending (LAD) artery (*arrow*) makes it in this patient very difficult to estimate the degree of stenosis and as such exclude obstructive coronary artery disease. The report should explicitly mention this, as further investigation may therefore be warranted.

decision-making on patient management on a per-patient basis.[5] It is based on the highest-grade coronary artery lesion documented by coronary CTA. Interpretation of the results with subsequent recommendations is further based on the clinical setting (stable vs. acute chest pain) under certain conditions. Implementation of this reporting system is not generalized and varies from center to center.

References

[1] Ghekiere O, Salgado R, Buls N, et al. Image quality in coronary CT angiography: challenges and technical solutions. Br J Radiol. 2017; 90(1072):20160567

[2] Pannu HK, Alvarez W, Jr, Fishman EK. Beta-blockers for cardiac CT: a primer for the radiologist. AJR Am J Roentgenol. 2006; 186(6) Suppl 2:S341–S345

[3] Carr JJ. Calcium scoring for cardiovascular computed tomography: how, when and why? Radiol Clin North Am. 2019; 57 (1):1–12

[4] Moss AJ, Williams MC, Newby DE, Nicol ED. The updated NICE guidelines: cardiac CT as the first-line test for coronary artery disease. Curr Cardiovasc Imaging Rep. 2017; 10(5):15

[5] Cury RC, Abbara S, Achenbach S, et al. Coronary artery disease–Reporting and Data System (CAD-RADS): an expert consensus document of SCCT, ACR and NASCI: endorsed by the ACC. JACC Cardiovasc Imaging. 2016; 9(9):1099–1113

48 Transcatheter Aortic Valve Implantation (TAVI)

Rodrigo Salgado, Marco Francone, and Ricardo P. J Budde

48.1 Template

Indication:
- Purpose of this procedure is preprocedural [aortic annulus and root sizing for TAVI/valve-in-valve implantation assessment]
- It [includes/does not include] evaluation of potential [endovascular/transaortic/supra-aortic/transapical] access routes

Native valve:
- The cuspidity of the native valve is [tricuspid/bicuspid/undefinable]
- Leaflet calcifications are [absent/mild/moderate/severe]
- Subvalvular calcifications are [present/absent] (add location when present)
- Agatston-score of leaflet calcifications: ___ (only indicated in discrepant Doppler echocardiography results)

Aortic annulus:
- Following measurements were performed in [systole/diastole]
- The quality of the measurements is [good/moderate/poor]
- Annular short- and long-axis diameter: __ × __ mm
- Annular perimeter: __ mm
- Annular area: __ mm^2
- Inner diameter of the degenerative prosthetic valve: __ mm (for valve-in-valve procedures)

Aortic sinus:
- Sinus height: __ mm
- Sinus width: __ mm
- Distance from annular plane to left main coronary ostium: __ mm
- Distance from annular plane to right coronary ostium: __ mm
- Diameter sinotubular junction: __ mm

Aorta:
Maximum cross-sectional diameter of the ascending aorta: [__ mm]
Aortic wall characteristics include (combinations of the following possible) [amount and distribution of calcification/presence of thrombus/presence of ulcerative plaques/aortic aneurysm or pseudo-aneurysm/dissection]
Access routes:

Artery	Luminal patency (patent/obstructive/occluded)	Minimal luminal diameter (mm)
Brachiocephalic artery		
Subclavian artery (left/right)		
Common iliac artery (left/right)		
External iliac artery (left/right)		
Common femoral artery (left/right)		

The apex of the left ventricle is [unremarkable/contains thrombus/(any other abnormal finding)]
Nonvascular findings:
There [are/are not] additional nonvascular findings which may influence the procedure and short-term outcome: (mention these findings)
There [are/are not] additional nonvascular findings which may influence the mid- and long-term short outcome: (mention these findings)

48.2 Stakeholders

Radiologists, interventional cardiologists, and cardiac surgeons involved in the preprocedural planning of TAVI candidates.

48.3 Pearls

- The aortic annulus is not a true anatomic structure, but a virtual ring formed by connecting the nadirs of the attachment sites of the aortic valve leaflets (at the basal portion of the sinus of Valsalva) (▸ Fig. 48.1). The annular plane of the aortic annulus is therefore defined

by connecting these three lowest insertion points of the aortic valve leaflets.
- The cross-sectional morphology of the aortic sinus is almost circular at the level of the sinotubular junction, but becomes more ellipsoid at the annular level (▸ Fig. 48.2). As such, the aortic annulus is very often not a circle but an oval structure with a short- and long-axis diameter. As such, computed tomography (CT) and ultrasound measurements do not compare well.
- The most commonly performed measurements of the aortic annulus are the cross-sectional short- and long-axis diameter, the annular perimeter, and area (▸ Fig. 48.3). As the annulus and aortic root have a double-oblique orientation, standard axial, sagittal, and coronal planes are not suitable for annular sizing.
- ECG-gated acquisition of the aortic root is essential. While a standard CT protocol for a routine examination of the coronary arteries can be used for the aortic root, several high-end CT systems have different approaches to achieve high-quality ECG-gated images.
- Systolic measurements of the aortic annulus are preferred.[1,2] However, when systolic images are of insufficient quality, measurements in diastole or in other phase of the cardiac cycle can be used for accurate measurements. The report must include mention of the cardiac phase in which the measurements were performed.
- Contrary to routine cardiac-CT examination, any premedication of the patient (e.g., use of beta-blockers or nitroglycerine) must be avoided as these are in general frail patients with often significant comorbidity.

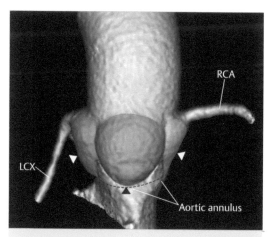

Fig. 48.1 The annulus is a virtual ring (*dashed line*), formed by connecting the nadirs of the attachment sites of the aortic valve leaflets at the basal portion of the sinuses of Valsalva (*arrowheads*).

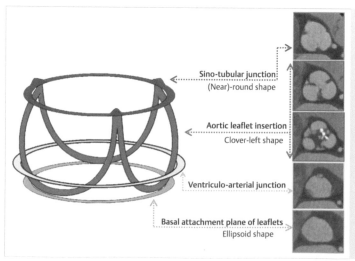

Fig. 48.2 The cross-sectional shape of the aortic root varies, with a (near) round shape at the level of the aortic sinus, evolving to a more oval shape at an annular level.

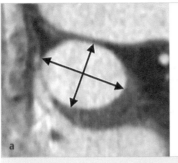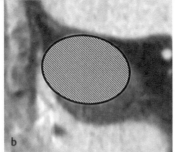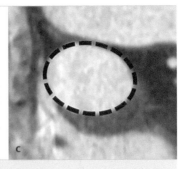

Fig. 48.3 The most commonly performed annular measurements are the cross-sectional long- and short-axis (a), area (b), and perimeter (c). These measurements must be performed in the correct double-oblique annular plane.

Table 48.1 Likelihood of having severe aortic valve stenosis based on MDCT quantification of valve leaflet calcifications using the Agatston-method

Agatston-score of aortic valve leaflets		
Likelihood of severe aortic valve stenosis	Men	Women
Score threshold	≥2000	≥1300

Source: Data from Pawade T et al 2019.[3]
Note: While not routinely executed, this approach may be problem-solving in equivocal low-flow/low-gradient cases in which Doppler ultrasound is unable to confirm a severe aortic valve stenosis.

Table 48.2 Proposal for visual grading of severity of aortic valve calcification

Semiquantitative pre-TAVI grading of valvular calcifications	
Absent	No calcifications
Mild	Small isolated focal spots not involving commissures and attachment sites
Moderate	Large confluent calcifications affecting two cusps or Small isolated focal spots at the level of all commissures and attachment sites
Severe	Large confluent calcifications affecting all cusps

Source: Adapted from Francone et al 2020.[2]

- Quantification of the aortic valve leaflets calcification is not a routine task but must currently be reserved for patients in which Doppler echocardiography is unable to confirm the presence of a severe aortic valve stenosis (e.g., in a low-flow, low-gradient situation). Some authors propose a likelihood of severe aortic valve stenosis depending on the obtained value[3] (▶ Table 48.1).
- For semiquantitative grading of valvular calcifications, a visual description as given in ▶ Table 48.2 is proposed.
- There are two types of currently clinically implemented transcatheter heart valves for treatment of aortic valve stenosis: balloon-expandable (e.g., SAPIEN series from Edwards Lifesciences) and self-expandable heart valves (e.g., EVOLUT range from Medtronic). Currently, only the balloon-expandable valve is available for a transapical approach.
- Optimal matching of a specific transcatheter valve size to a patient's anatomy is essential in order to avoid pre- and postprocedural complications. However, sizing algorithms differ between the types of transcatheter valves, and also between different versions of these valves. Consult with the vendor for valve-specific guidelines.
- Presence of a bicuspid valve is not a contraindication but may increase procedural complexity and has been associated with a high rate of postprocedural pacemaker implantation.[4]

References

[1] Blanke P, Weir-McCall JR, Achenbach S, et al. Computed tomography imaging in the context of transcatheter aortic valve implantation (TAVI)/transcatheter aortic valve replacement (TAVR): an expert consensus document of the Society of Cardiovascular Computed Tomography. J Cardiovasc Comput Tomogr. 2019; 13(1):1–20

[2] Francone M, Budde R, Bremerich J, et al. CT and MR imaging prior to transcatheter aortic valve implantation: standardization of scanning protocols, measurements and reporting. A consensus document by the European Society of Cardiovascular Radiology (ESCR). Eur Radiol. 2020; 30(5):2627–2650

[3] Pawade T, Sheth T, Guzzetti E. et al. Why and how to measure aortic valve calcification in patients with aortic stenosis. J Am Coll Cardiol Cardiovasc Imaging 2019 12(9):1835–1848

[4] Jilaihawi H, Chen M, Webb J, et al. A bicuspid aortic valve imaging classification for the TAVR era. JACC Cardiovasc Imaging. 2016; 9(10):1145–1158

49 Cardiac MR Examination: Cardiomyopathy in an Adult Patient

Jean-Nicolas Dacher

49.1 Template

Technical quality:
The quality of the examination is [excellent/good/poor]
Anatomy:
The great vessels of the mediastinum are [normal/abnormal]. (If abnormal, describe anomaly.)
There is [normal/increased] increased pericardial fluid. (If increased, quantify in mm fluid thickness.)
The thickness of the pericardium is [normal/increased]. (If increased, quantify in mm thickness.)
Myocardial segments have a [normal/increased] thickness
- If yes, provide additional information:
  - Diffuse/segmental; symmetric/asymmetric
  - Indicate thickened segments (Bull's eye, ▶ Fig. 49.1)
  - Presence of edema: yes/no (on STIR, T2-weighted images)
    - If yes, precise involved segments
  - Quantify thickening (reminder: do not include trabeculations; no hypertrophy if myocardium < 13 mm in diastole; hypertrophy if > 13 mm; gray zone in between)
    - Precise possible right ventricle (RV) involvement
    - Precise if atypical left ventricle (LV) appearance
      - Clefts
      - Abnormal papillary muscles
      - Abnormal mitral valve length
      - > 30 mm for anterior leaflet
      - > 17 mm for posterior leaflet
  - LV/RV noncompaction
  - Thrombus
  - Subaortic obstruction

Function:
Following measurements were taken:

Ejection fraction LV (%)		
Ejection fraction RV (%)		
LV mass at end-diastole (absolute and indexed[a], g and g/m^2)	.../...	

Volumes		
Anatomy	Diastole (absolute, mL)/ (indexed[a], mL/m^2)	Systole (absolute, mL)/(indexed[a], mL/m^2)
Left ventricle	.../...	.../...
Right ventricle	.../...	.../...
Left atrium[b]	N/A	.../...

[a]Indexed to body mass area.
[b]Measured at systole (0.85 × 4C view LA area × 2C view LA area/shortest LA length).

Wall kinetics are [normal/abnormal]
- If abnormal, specify additional details:
  - Global hypokinesia
  - Focal hypokinesia/akinesia
  - Focal dyskinesia (RV should be carefully examined in the context of suspected ARVC/D)
  - Asynchrony

Mapping (optional):
Native T1-mapping is [normal/increased/decreased]
- If abnormal, precise diffuse/segmental

Extracellular volume is [normal/abnormal]
- If abnormal, precise diffuse/segmental
- ECV additional info
  - Mean%
  - If segmental anomaly, precise segment

Native T2-mapping is [normal/increased]
- If increased, precise diffuse or segmental

Native T2* is [normal/decreased].
Perfusion:
A [rest/stress] perfusion examination was performed. The result is [normal/abnormal]
- If abnormal, precise
  - Number of segments
  - Coronary artery territory (Bull's eye, ▶ Fig. 49.1)
  - Subendocardial/transmural involvement

Delayed enhancement is [normal/abnormal]
- If abnormal, precise
  - Number of segments
  - Coronary artery territory (Bull's eye, ▶ Fig. 49.1)
  - Subendocardial/midwall/subepicardial involvement

49.2 Stakeholders

Radiologists and cardiologists.

49.3 Pearls

- Cardiac magnetic resonance (MR) imaging is currently the cornerstone examination in any patient with a primitive cardiomyopathy (CM). A typical MR protocol is given in ▶ Table 49.1, with the current American Heart Association classification[1] in ▶ Fig. 49.2. A model for left ventricular myocardial segmentation can be found in ▶ Fig. 49.1.[2]
- In the context of dilated CM, differentiating ischemic from nonischemic cardiopathy is of primary importance (among others, the presence/absence of segmental subendocardial delayed enhancement) (▶ Fig. 49.3).
- In the context of hypertrophic CM, cardiac MR provides arguments for genetic disease

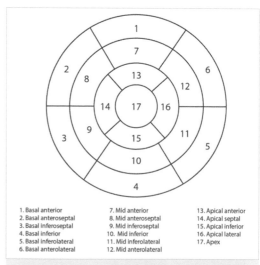

1. Basal anterior	7. Mid anterior	13. Apical anterior
2. Basal anteroseptal	8. Mid anteroseptal	14. Apical septal
3. Basal inferoseptal	9. Mid inferoseptal	15. Apical inferior
4. Basal inferior	10. Mid inferior	16. Apical lateral
5. Basal inferolateral	11. Mid inferolateral	17. Apex
6. Basal anterolateral	12. Mid anterolateral	

Fig. 49.1 Left ventricular myocardial segmentation, 17 segment model. (Reproduced with permission from Cerqueira MD, Weissman NJ, Dilsizian V, et al 2002.[2])

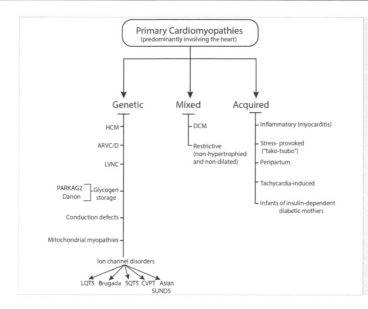

Fig. 49.2 American Heart Association classification of cardiomyopathies. (Reproduced with permission McKenna WJ, Maron BJ and Thiene G, 2017.[1])

Table 49.1 Overview of typical MR sequences performed in the work-up of a patient with a suspected or known cardiomyopathy

Typical magnetic resonance (MR) sequence protocol

Scout views

CINE steady state free precession (SSFP)

Axial multislice coverage of the chest
Stack of short axis (SA) views covering the whole ventricles
4-chamber view (4C-horizontal long axis)
Left ventricle (LV) vertical long axis
Right ventricle (RV) vertical long axis
3-chamber view
Left ventricular outflow tract (LVOT) view
SA view of the aortic root

STIR

4C view
3 SA views (base, midventricle, apex)

Mapping (optional)

3 SA views (base, midventricle, apex): T1 and T2 mapping
Midventricular SA view: T2* mapping

Perfusion imaging

First pass
Optional stress perfusion imaging (adenosine/Regadenoson)

Delayed enhancement

T1-weighted images 10 min after gadolinium injection

Optional

Repeat T1-mapping sequence at 10 min postinjection
Infer extracellular volume from nonenhanced and enhanced T1 maps

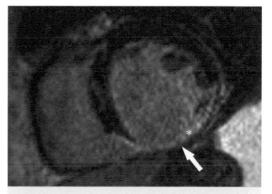

Fig. 49.3 Ischemic cardiomyopathy with postinfarct thinning of the inferior wall (*arrow*). The delayed-enhancement on T1-weighted images after intravenous contrast administration indicates scar tissue (*asterisk*).

(asymmetry, fibrosis, obstruction) or orients toward a differential diagnosis (hypertension, Fabry disease, amyloidosis, aortic stenosis, and others).

- Arrhythmogenic right ventricular dysplasia/cardiomyopathy is a genetic disease inducing a risk of sudden death. The diagnosis is based on multiple criteria including cardiac MR analysis of kinetics, RV ejection fraction, and volumes.[3]
- T1-, T2-, and T2* mapping techniques are increasingly important in the evaluation of primitive cardiomyopathies. Basically, native T1 and ECV values increase in myocardial fibrosis, increased T2 is a marker of edema/inflammation (myocarditis).[4] T2* is decreased in iron overload. Interestingly, native T1 is significantly decreased

in Fabry disease and significantly increased in amyloidosis.

- Cardiac MR is efficient in differentiating constrictive vs. restrictive cardiomyopathy. Presence/absence of a thickened pericardium (a challenging situation for echocardiography) is easily diagnosed on MR.
- In the absence of confounding factors (atrial fibrillation, mitral valve regurgitation), a dilated left atrium with nondilated left ventricle argues for diastolic dysfunction[5] and restrictive cardiomyopathy.

References

[1] McKenna WJ, Maron BJ, Thiene G. Classification, epidemiology, and global burden of cardiomyopathies. Circ Res. 2017; 121(7):722–730

[2] Cerqueira MD, Weissman NJ, Dilsizian V, et al. American Heart Association Writing Group on Myocardial Segmentation and Registration for Cardiac Imaging. Standardized myocardial segmentation and nomenclature for tomographic imaging of the heart. A statement for healthcare professionals from the Cardiac Imaging Committee of the Council on Clinical Cardiology of the American Heart Association. Circulation. 2002; 105(4):539–542

[3] Marcus FI, McKenna WJ, Sherrill D, et al. Diagnosis of arrhythmogenic right ventricular cardiomyopathy/dysplasia: proposed modification of the Task Force Criteria. Eur Heart J. 2010; 31(7):806–814

[4] Ferreira VM, Schulz-Menger J, Holmvang G, et al. Cardiovascular magnetic resonance in nonischemic myocardial inflammation: expert recommendations. J Am Coll Cardiol. 2018; 72(24):3158–3176

[5] Caudron J, Fares J, Bauer F, Dacher JN. Evaluation of left ventricular diastolic function with cardiac MR imaging. Radiographics. 2011; 31(1):239–259

50 Abdominal Aortic Aneurysm (AAA): Postprocedural Surveillance

Rodrigo Salgado

50.1 Template

Indication and CT protocol:
- Purpose of this procedure is the postprocedural surveillance of an AAA after [endovascular/open surgical] repair
- The CT examination has been performed [with/without] intravenous contrast administration

Aneurysm location and morphology:
- The aneurysm is located in the [infrarenal/suprarenal/infra- and suprarenal] aorta
- Its morphology is [fusiform/saccular]
- Extension into the [left/right] common iliac artery is [present/absent]

Measurements:
Following measurements were performed:
- Maximal cross-sectional edge-to-edge diameter of the treated aneurysm: __ mm
- Maximal sac volume: __ mL
- The treated AAA size is [stable/has increased] compared with the measurement on the previous examination of (insert date), [with an amount of __mm or mL]
- The gross morphology of the treated AAA has [not changed/changed]

Graft position and patency:
- The distance from the lower edge of the lowest renal ostium to the proximal edge of the aneurysmal sac is __mm
- The position of the stent-graft is [stable/has migrated]. (When migrated, provide distance of proximal edge to lowest renal artery.)
- The [endograft/surgical aortoiliac graft/surgical aortofemoral graft] is [patent/obstructed/occluded]
- Endoleakage is [present/absent] with a type [I (a,b)/II/III/IV/V/undetermined] endoleak at (specify location)

Luminal and wall assessment:
There are [no/known/new] signs of [extensive thrombus/ulcerative plaques/infection/inflammation/dissection/pseudoaneurysm/other] along the [endovascular grafts/surgical anastomoses]. (Specify detailed location.)
The [are/are no] signs of acutely increased rupture risk. (When present, provide additional details.)
Free abdominal fluid is [present/absent]
Entry sites evaluation:
The [left/right] common femoral artery has a [normal/abnormal] postprocedural appearance, [with/without] regional complications
(When applicable) The following complications are now present at the [left/right] common femoral artery: [pseudoaneurysm/abscess/collection/sign of infection or inflammation/arteriovenous fistula]
Nonvascular findings:
- There [are/are not] additional nonvascular findings which may influence the immediate and short-term outcome: (mention these findings when present)
- There [are/are not] additional nonvascular findings which may influence the mid- and long-term short outcome: (mention these findings when present)

50.2 Stakeholders

General and cardiovascular, interventional radiologist and vascular surgeons involved in the postprocedural surveillance of abdominal aneurysms.

50.3 Pearls

- The main goals of postprocedural surveillance can be found in ▸ Table 50.1. Successful exclusion of the AAA from the systemic circulation eliminates aneurysm growth and risk of rupture (▸ Fig. 50.1 and ▸ Fig. 50.2).

Table 50.1 Targets of imaging surveillance

Evaluation of stent-graft patency and structural integrity
Size assessment of the sealed aneurysmal sac
Detection and characterization of endoleaks
Assessment of positional changes of the graft (e.g., graft migration)
Long-term follow-up of graft durability

- Unenhanced computed tomography (CT) may be considered for size follow-up in uncomplicated cases as long as postprocedural dimensions of the excluded AAA remain stable (volumetric change less than 2%) or diminish compared with preprocedural examinations. It is also helpful in distinguishing calcified thrombotic material from endoleakage (▸ Fig. 50.1).
- In other cases, and also the method of choice in many centers, contrast-enhanced CT with intravenous contrast administration will deliver the most complete assessment.[1,2] Contrast-enhanced magnetic resonance (MR) can also be used when executed properly, although it has a higher procedural complexity and is less practical for taking longitudinal measurements along curved vascular paths. In case of renal dysfunction, an unenhanced CT or MR examination can be considered. Finally, recent studies suggest a comparable accuracy for contrast-enhanced ultrasound.

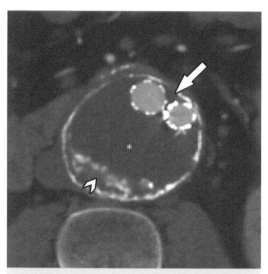

Fig. 50.1 Axial contrast-enhanced computed tomography (CT) image after successful endovascular aneurysm repair (EVAR). The aneurysm is excluded from the normal circulation by the endovascular stent-grafts (*arrow*), with subsequent thrombosis of the original aneurysmal sac (*asterisk*). On occasion, old calcifications in thrombotic material can be found within the aneurysmal sac, which must not be confused for leakage. Comparison with previous examinations or inclusion of an unenhanced acquisition is often problem-solving.

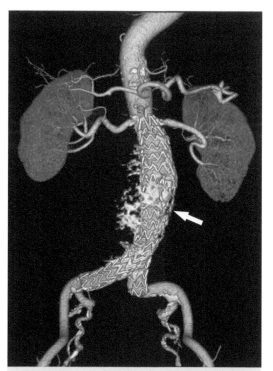

Fig. 50.2 Volume-rendered computed tomography (CT) image after successful endovascular aneurysm repair (EVAR). The endovascular graft (*arrow*) has a normal position, extending from the level of the renal arteries to the common iliac arteries. Remaining calcifications can be seen in the thrombosed native aneurysmal sac (compare with ▸ Fig. 50.1).

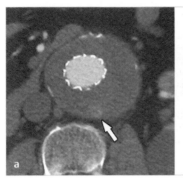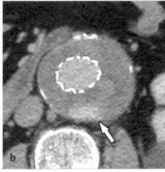

Fig. 50.3(a, b) Type II endoleak in a patient after endovascular aneurysm repair (EVAR) of an intrarenal abdominal aneurysm. In the initial arterial contrast phase, only a faint dense blush is visible posteriorly within the aneurysmal sac. On the delayed-phase acquisition, this endoleak is much more noticeable due to further retrograde filling of the aneurysmal sac, in this case through a paralumbar artery.

Table 50.2 Types of endoleaks and their significance

Type of endoleak	Origin of leak	Intervention needed	Percentage
I	Ia: proximal end of endograft Ib: distal end of endograft	Urgent repair	12%
II	Retrograde flow in excluded AAA sac from connecting arteries (IMA, lumbar arteries)	Further surveillance without intervention in stable dimensions. May resolve spontaneously. Repair in case of size increase	76%
III	IIIa: endograft modular component leak IIIb: endograft fabric leak	Urgent repair, although rare with current modern endografts	3
IV	Increased graft porosity	No or rarely intervention needed	3
Indeterminate	Often unknown. Expanding aneurysmal sac without identifiable cause	Decision on a case-by-case basis. Consider MR for detection of CT-occult endoleaks	6%

Abbreviations: AAA, abdominal aortic aneurysm; CT, computed tomography; IMA, inferior mesenteric artery; MR, magnetic resonance.
Source: Adapted from Partovi et al 2018; Guo et al 2016; Chaikof et al 2018.[2,4,5]

- Every contrast-enhanced CT must include an arterial phase and a delayed-phase after 120 seconds to increase detection of endoleaks. Endoleaks are defined as persistent blood flow within the inadequately excluded aneurysmal sac (▶ Fig. 50.3(a, b)). Several studies have indicated a higher sensitivity of MR to detect endoleaks in equivocal cases of increasing aneurysmal sac size without a clear etiology on CT.[3]
- Depending on the renal function, a combination of alternating imaging modalities with and without intravenous contrast administration may be considered.
- Five types of endoleaks have been described (▶ Table 50.2).[2] The overall presence of endoleaks have been recently estimated to be about 26%, with type II being most common.[4] Type II leaks are low-flow leaks, may resolve spontaneously, and often do not require intervention. Only when the size of the aneurysm expands more than 5 mm, an intervention may be considered on a case-by-case basis, also contemplating other patient comorbidities and local center policies.
- In contrast, type I and III are considered high-flow endoleaks, with faster progression and increasing risk for postimplant rupture.[5] As such, urgent intervention is required upon detection.
- Postprocedural surveillance is typically performed with contrast-enhanced CT at 1, 6, and 12 months after the procedure. Lifelong annual follow-up is recommended, as endoleaks can occur at any moment from the immediate postprocedural period to decades later.
- Similarly to preprocedural AAA sizing, measurements must be obtained in a plane perpendicular to the long axis of the investigated aortic segment and performed between the outer

edges of the aneurysm. Volumetric assessment of the aneurysmal sac has also been advocated for follow-up, although in practice rarely performed for practical reasons.

References

[1] Bryce Y, Rogoff P, Romanelli D, Reichle R. Endovascular repair of abdominal aortic aneurysms: vascular anatomy, device selection, procedure, and procedure-specific complications. Radiographics. 2015; 35(2):593–615

[2] Partovi S, Trischman T, Rafailidis V, et al. Multimodality imaging assessment of endoleaks post-endovascular aortic repair. Br J Radiol. 2018; 91(1087):20180013

[3] Habets J, Zandvoort HJ, Reitsma JB, et al. Magnetic resonance imaging is more sensitive than computed tomography angiography for the detection of endoleaks after endovascular abdominal aortic aneurysm repair: a systematic review. Eur J Vasc Endovasc Surg. 2013; 45(4):340–350

[4] Guo Q, Zhao J, Huang B, et al. A systematic review of ultrasound or magnetic resonance imaging compared with computed tomography for endoleak detection and aneurysm diameter measurement after endovascular aneurysm repair. J Endovasc Ther. 2016; 23(6):936–943

[5] Chaikof EL, Dalman RL, Eskandari MK, et al. The Society for Vascular Surgery practice guidelines on the care of patients with an abdominal aortic aneurysm. J Vasc Surg. 2018; 67 (1):2–77.e2

51 Abdominal Aortic Aneurysm (AAA): Preprocedural Evaluation

Rodrigo Salgado

51.1 Template

Indication:
Purpose of this procedure is the [work-up of a newly found AAA/follow-up of a known AAA]
Aneurysm location and morphology:
The aneurysm is located in the [infrarenal/suprarenal/infra- and suprarenal] aorta
Its morphology is [fusiform/saccular]
Extension into the [left/right] common iliac artery is [present/absent]
Measurements:
Following cross-sectional measurements were performed (edge-to-edge diameter):
Suprarenal aorta: __ mm
Aorta at the level of the renal arteries: __ mm
Infrarenal aorta: __ mm
Right common iliac artery: __ mm
Right external iliac artery: __ mm
Left common iliac artery: __ mm
Right external iliac artery: __ mm
Distance measurements, from the lower edge of the lowest renal ostium
to the proximal edge of the AAA (aortic neck): __ mm
to the distal edge of the AAA: __ mm
to the aortoiliac bifurcation: __ mm
to the right iliac bifurcation: __ mm
to the left iliac bifurcation: __ mm
The aortic neck is [patent/obstructive] with [acceptable wall delineation/significant atherosclerosis]
There is [unremarkable/marked] tortuosity of the aortic neck angle. (Provide details when marked.)
There is [unremarkable/marked] tortuosity of the [left/right/bilateral] aortoiliac axis. (Provide details when marked.)
(When applicable) The AAA size is [stable/has increased] compared with the measurement on the previous examination of (insert date), [with an amount of __ mm]
The gross morphology of the AAA has [not changed/changed]
Luminal and wall assessment:
There are [no/known/newly found] signs of [extensive thrombus/ulcerative plaques/infection/inflammation] in the [aorta/right iliac arteries/left iliac arteries] (specify detailed location)
The [are/are no] signs of acutely increased rupture risk. (When present, add the following) Signs of acutely increased rupture risk include [periaortic fat infiltration/high-attenuating crescent sign/draped aorta sign/interruption of ring of intimal calcification/other]
Free abdominal fluid is [present/absent]
Access routes for endovascular treatment:
The lumen of the [left/right] [common/external] artery is [patent/obstructive/occluded] with a minimal diameter of [__ mm]
The lumen of the [left/right] [common femoral artery is [patent/obstructive/occluded] with a minimal diameter of [__ mm]
Nonvascular findings:
There [are/are not] additional nonvascular findings which may influence the immediate and short-term outcome: (mention these findings when present)
There [are/are not] additional nonvascular findings which may influence the mid- and long-term short outcome: (mention these findings when present)

51.2 Stakeholders

General and cardiovascular radiologists, interventional radiologists, and vascular surgeons involved in the preprocedural planning and surveillance of abdominal aneurysms.

51.3 Pearls

- An abdominal aortic diameter of at least 3 cm is considered to be aneurysmal, being often more than 2 standard deviations above the mean diameter for men.[1,2] However, there is no consensus on the actual definition of an abdominal aortic aneurysm (AAA).[3]

- Most atherosclerotic aneurysms are fusiform, expanding in an equal fashion in all directions (▶ Fig. 51.1). A saccular aneurysm has a more asymmetric expansion favoring one side. A true aneurysm involves all layers of the aortic wall (intima, media, adventitia). They can be fusiform or saccular.

- However, the term *saccular* must not be confused with a pseudoaneurysm, which is not composed of all layers of the aortic wall; the outer layer is often formed of fibrous material. Pseudoaneurysms are often the result of infection or local trauma, and present frequently as a focal outpouching of the aorta with a saccular morphology and concomitant infectious/inflammatory signs. Contrary to atherosclerotic aneurysms, their rupture risk is unrelated to size, with often fast growth and fatal outcome if untreated (▶ Fig. 51.2). The usually employed term "mycotic aneurysm" is a misnomer, as infectious pseudoaneurysm is commonly caused by bacteria (*Salmonella* or *Staphylococcus aureus*).

- An AAA can contain a varying amount of luminal (often semicircular) thrombus, which may also include calcified components (▶ Fig. 51.1). These must not be confused with intramural penetration of blood.

- While ultrasound is useful for screening and surveillance of AAA, many centers use CT for at least the initial evaluation of a previously unknown AAA, benefiting from the superior image quality and accurate assessment of its characteristics. Depending on the characteristics of the AAA and patient (e.g., obesity), the choice between ultrasound and CT is then evaluated for

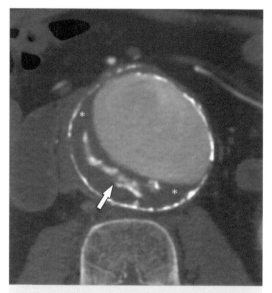

Fig. 51.1 Contrast-enhanced computed tomography (CT) of a fusiform infrarenal abdominal aortic aneurysm (AAA). Note the semicircular intraluminal thrombus (*asterisk*), and the presence of amorphous calcified thrombotic material (*arrow*). This must not be confused with intramural blood penetration. An unenhanced CT acquisition of comparison with previous examinations is often problem-solving.

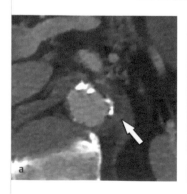
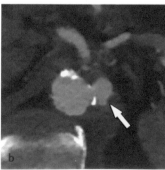

Fig. 51.2 Rapid progression of an infectious (*Salmonella* sp.) pseudoaneurysm in the suprarenal aorta. On day 1 **(a)**, only a discrete irregular bulge is noted along the left side of the aortic wall, with limited soft tissue infiltration. Subsequent follow-up on day 5 **(b)** illustrate the rapid progression of this pseudoaneurysm, which prompted an urgent intervention. Note the normal intrinsic dimensions of the aorta, underlining the fact that rupture risk of a pseudoaneurysm is not related to aortic size.

further follow-up, sometimes alternating between these imaging modalities.

- In case of renal dysfunction, an unenhanced CT or MR examination can be considered.
- Measurements must be obtained in a plane perpendicular to the long axis of the investigated aortic segment and performed between the outer edges of the aneurysm. Given the often-tortuous aspect of the aortoiliac arteries, standard axial, sagittal, or coronal planes are not adequate for correct sizing of an AAA.
- In a typical atherosclerotic aneurysm, rupture risk increases with diameter (▶ Fig. 51.3). When the diameter is 5 cm or more, the annular rupture risk is estimated at 11% per year, increasing to 25% annually for an AAA size of ≥ 6 cm.[1] Reimbursement modalities vary on the size of the AAA and speed of growth across countries. In general, a threshold of about 5 cm is generally accepted as an indication for intervention. However, lower thresholds may be appropriate for women, as studies indicate rupture of AAA in women with a greater frequency than men at all size intervals, with a fourfold increased frequency of rupture at < 5.5 cm.[4]
- The preferred treatment of an AAA is endovascular aneurysm repair (EVAR), a technique where the aneurysm is excluded from the systemic circulation using an endograft with iliac extensions endovascularly delivered through the common femoral arteries. As such, preprocedural knowledge of the exact anatomic dimensions of the involved arteries and the distances between bifurcations is critical for the correct choice of graft size, graft length and the resulting procedural success (▶ Fig. 51.4).
- An important point to consider here is the distance between the lowest ostium of the renal arteries and the proximal origin of the AAA, as an unaffected (free of extensive calcification and thrombus) landing zone of about 1 to 1.5 cm is general accepted as a minimum for safe procedural execution (▶ Fig. 51.4). In case of a juxtarenal AAA (no proximal landing zone), extensive angulation or other factors increasing procedural risk, more complex endovascular techniques, or open surgical repair may be considered at increased procedural risk.

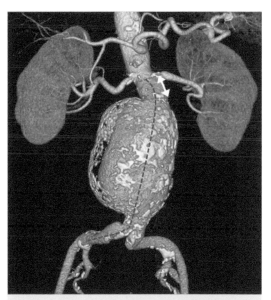

Fig. 51.4 Volume-rendered contrast-enhanced CT image of an infrarenal abdominal aortic aneurysm (AAA). An unaffected aortic neck (*double arrow*) of 1 to 1.5 cm length is an important prerequisite for endovascular treatment as it acts as the proximal landing zone for the endovascular graft. Also, other anatomic cross-sectional dimensions and longitudinal distances (*dotted lines*) along arterial pathways at several anatomical reference points must be delivered in order to safely plan endovascular treatment.

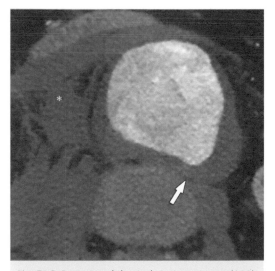

Fig. 51.3 Rupturing abdominal aortic aneurysm (AAA) of 7 cm cross-section diameter. The draped aorta sign is illustrated as the aorta follows the anterior contour of the spine on the left side (*arrow*). Extensive periaortic hemorrhage (*asterisk*) is also clearly present.

References

[1] Chaikof EL, Dalman RL, Eskandari MK, et al. The Society for Vascular Surgery practice guidelines on the care of patients with an abdominal aortic aneurysm. J Vasc Surg. 2018; 67 (1):2–77.e2

[2] Golledge J. Abdominal aortic aneurysm: update on pathogenesis and medical treatments. Nat Rev Cardiol. 2019; 16 (4):225–242

[3] Sakalihasan N, Michel JB, Katsargyris A, et al. Abdominal aortic aneurysms. Nat Rev Dis Primers. 2018; 4(1):34

[4] Skibba AA, Evans JR, Hopkins SP, et al. Reconsidering gender relative to risk of rupture in the contemporary management of abdominal aortic aneurysms. J Vasc Surg. 2015; 62 (6):1429–1436

52 Coronary Arteries Calcium Quantitative CT Score

Daniela M. Tridente and Diana Litmanovich

52.1 Template

Findings:
Agatston score:
The total (aggregate) calcium score using the AJ 130 method is [ ]. Total volume score of [ ]
[ ]% of similar patients have less coronary artery calcium
Individual major vessel AJ 130 scores are: LM:[ ]; LAD:[ ]; LCX:[ ]; RCA:[ ]
Cardiac morphology:
Heart size is [normal/enlarged] with [no/mild/moderate/large] pericardial effusion. There is conventional anatomy of the coronary arteries
Great vessels measurements (mm): ascending aorta: [ ]; descending aorta: [ ]; main pulmonary artery: [ ]
Extracoronary calcifications:
- [No/mild/moderate/severe] aortic valve calcification
- [No/mild/moderate/severe] thoracic aorta calcification
- [No/mild/moderate/severe] mitral annular calcification

Extracardiac findings:
- The thyroid is unremarkable
- No mediastinal or hilar lymphadenopathy
- Lungs are clear bilaterally, with patent airways. No suspicious nodules
- No worrisome osseous lesions

Impression and recommendations:
Total calcium score of [ ]
CAC-DRS category A [0/1/2/3]/N [1/2/3]
(A—risk category based on Agatston score/N—number of coronary arteries with calcifications)
CAC score risk: CAC-DRS
[0—very low risk, statin generally not recommended
1—mildly increased risk, moderate intensity statin recommended
2—moderately increased risk, moderate-to-high intensity statin + 81 mg ASA recommended
3—moderately increased risk, moderate-to-high intensity statin + 81 mg ASA recommended]

52.2 Stakeholders

Radiologists, cardiologists, cardiac surgeons, interventional cardiologists, primary care physicians, nuclear medicine physicians, and pulmonologists.

52.3 Pearls

- The inflammation associated to the formation of atherosclerotic plaques causes dysregulation of the mechanisms that control tissue concentration of calcium and phosphorous. The resultant calcium-phosphate crystals aggregate and, when they *exceed 0.2 mm in size, they become visible on computed tomography (CT).*
- Coronary artery calcifications (CAC) can be assessed either through visual estimation (reserved for nongated CTs) or Agatston scoring (ECG-gated or non-ECG-gated CTs).
- *Calcium score should not be performed on patients with stents and bypasses*: the presence of these already infer the existence of coronary artery disease (CAD) and calcium score would be overestimated due to the high density of the stents.
- High heart rates may cause motion artifacts and blurring of images, possibly creating false increase in Agatston score. Agatston scoring is not recommended if heart rate is above 80 beats per minute. Beta-blockers can be considered for rate control in selected patients.
- It is important to distinguish between coronary and noncoronary calcifications when calculating the calcium score. *Noncoronary calcifications*

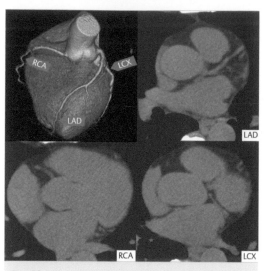

Fig. 52.1 Coronary artery calcification (CAC) 0—unenhanced axial slice of cardiac computed tomography (CT) with no calcifications in any coronary arteries. LAD, left anterior descending artery; LCX, left circumflex artery; RCA, right coronary artery.

that should be excluded from the score: aortic root, mitral annulus, or pericardial calcifications.

- After assessment, CAC should be graded 0–3 (▶ Fig. 52.1, ▶ Fig. 52.2, ▶ Fig. 52.3, and ▶ Fig. 52.4). If CAC ≥ 1, modifier N (number of vessels with CAC) should be added. The modifier does not influence the category; however, it may alter the aggressiveness of treatment. This modification has also proven to provide better stratification of risk for cardiovascular disease (CVD), coronary heart disease, and all-cause death.

- Patients with higher CAC scores are at greater risk of fatal and nonfatal myocardial infarction. CAC-DRS category 0 has shown to be the strongest negative risk marker in clinical practice for identifying patients with very low 10-year risk for CVD (▶ Table 52.1).

- CAC is a tombstone of disease and not necessarily related to the plaque most likely to cause atherosclerotic CVD as it may represent an inactive atheroma, unlikely to break free and embolize to distant vessels.

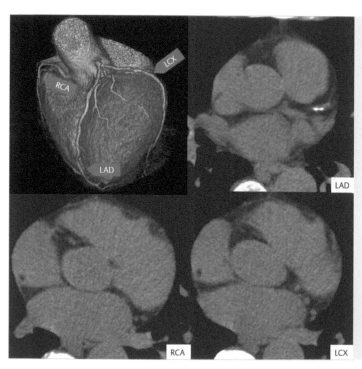

Fig. 52.2 Coronary artery calcification (CAC) 1—unenhanced axial slice of cardiac computed tomography (CT) with punctuate calcifications in the LAD and none in the other coronary arteries (Agatston 78—A1 N1). LAD, left anterior descending artery; LCX, left circumflex artery; RCA, right coronary artery.

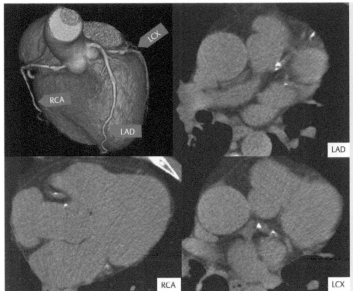

Fig. 52.3 Coronary artery calcification (CAC) 2—unenhanced axial slice of cardiac computed tomography (CT) with linear calcifications in all coronary arteries (Agatston 246—A2 N3). LAD, left anterior descending artery; LCX, left circumflex artery; RCA, right coronary artery.

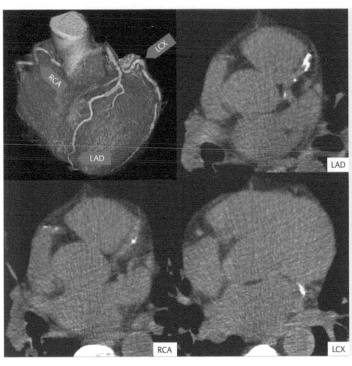

Fig. 52.4 Coronary artery calcification (CAC) 3—unenhanced axial slice of cardiac computed tomography (CT) with long calcified atherosclerotic plaques in the LAD and linear calcified plaques in the other coronary arteries (Agatston 478—A3 N3). LAD, left anterior descending artery; LCX, left circumflex artery; RCA, right coronary artery.

Table 52.1 Agatston score is a base for CAC-DRS category and determines risk classifications and treatment recommendations

CAC-DRS[a]: CAC score–risk treatment recommendation
CAC-DRS 0: 0 very low risk, statin generally not recommended[b]
CAC-DRS 1: 1–99 mildly increased risk, moderate intensity statin
CAC-DRS 2: 100–299 moderately increased risk, moderate to high intensity statin + ASA 81mg
CAC-DRS 3: > moderately to severely increased risk, high intensity statin + ASA 81mg

Source: Adapted from Hecht et al 2018.[1]
[a]Modifier N (number of vessels with CAC) does not influence the category; however, it may alter the aggressiveness of treatment. Thus, it should be reported if CAC > 0.
[b]Excluding familial hypercholesterolemia.
Abbreviation: ASA, acetylsalicylic acid; CAC, coronary artery calcification(s); CAC-DRS, Coronary artery calcium data and reporting system.

- CAC scoring is a screening tool. Symptomatic patients with negative scores should be further evaluated with coronary CT angiography (CTA) to definitively rule out noncalcified atherosclerotic disease.

Suggested Readings

Calcium scoring is reported using the interactive MESA form (www.mesanhlbi.org/CACReference.aspx) and graded using the CAC-DRS classification. J Cardiovasc Comput Tomogr. 2018; 12(3):185–191

Dzaye O, Dudum R, Mirbolouk M, et al. Validation of the Coronary Artery Calcium Data and Reporting System (CAC-DRS): dual importance of CAC score and CAC distribution from the coronary artery calcium (CAC) consortium. J Cardiovasc Comput Tomogr. 2020; 14(1):12–17

Hecht HS, Blaha MJ, Kazerooni EA, et al. CAC-DRS: Coronary Artery Calcium Data and Reporting System. An expert consensus document of the Society of Cardiovascular Computed Tomography (SCCT). J Cardiovasc Comput Tomogr. 2018; 12(3):185–191

Strauss HW, Nakahara T, Narula N, Narula J. Vascular calcification: the evolving relationship of vascular calcification to major acute coronary events. J Nucl Med. 2019; 60(9):1207–1212

van der Werf NR, Willemink MJ, Willems TP, Vliegenthart R, Greuter MJW, Leiner T. Influence of heart rate on coronary calcium scores: a multi-manufacturer phantom study. Int J Cardiovasc Imaging. 2018; 34(6):959–966

Williams MC, Moss A, Dweck M, et al. Standardized reporting systems for computed tomography coronary angiography and calcium scoring: a real-world validation of CAD-RADS and CAC-DRS in patients with stable chest pain. J Cardiovasc Comput Tomogr. 2020; 14(1):3–11

53 Fractional Flow Reserve (FFR) CT for Coronary CTA

Daniela M. Tridente and Diana Litmanovich

53.1 Template

Findings:
Left main artery: [no/focal/diffuse] [calcified/noncalcified/mixed] atherosclerotic plaque in the [proximal/mid/distal] [name vessel/branch] with a [low/borderline/high] likelihood of flow-limiting stenosis due to an FFR value of [ ]
Lad and branches: [no/focal/diffuse] [calcified/noncalcified/mixed] atherosclerotic plaque in the [proximal/mid/distal] [name vessel/branch] with a [low/borderline/high] likelihood of flow-limiting stenosis due to an FFR value of [ ]
LCX and branches: [no/focal/diffuse] [calcified/noncalcified/mixed] atherosclerotic plaque in the [proximal/mid/distal] [name vessel/branch] with a [low/borderline/high] likelihood of flow-limiting stenosis due to an FFR value of [ ]
RCA and branches: [no/focal/diffuse] [calcified/noncalcified/mixed] atherosclerotic plaque in the [proximal/mid/distal] [name vessel/branch] with a [low/borderline/high] likelihood of flow-limiting stenosis due to an FFR value of [ ]

Impression:
FFR CT values suggestive of [no/low likelihood/borderline likelihood/high likelihood] hemodynamically significant stenoses in [*name vessels*]

Recommendation(s):*
- In patients with *no evidence of flow-limiting stenoses*, consider medical management and risk factor modification
- In patients with *low likelihood of flow-limiting stenoses*, consider statin therapy as tolerated and risk factor modification
- In patients with *borderline likelihood of flow-limiting stenoses*, consider intensive medical therapy (statin, ASA, and beta-blocker as tolerated). Consider invasive coronary angiography with invasive FFR in selected cases
- In patients with *high likelihood of flow-limiting stenoses*, intensive medical therapy is recommended. Consider invasive angiography with invasive FFR in selected cases

FFR CT is a FDA-cleared noninvasive technique for defining the probability of flow-limiting coronary stenoses that correlates with invasive FFR measurements. As with all testing, clinical correlation is advised
* Recommendations should be discussed and approved with the referring physicians and, ideally, should be center specific.

53.2 Stakeholders

Radiologists, cardiologists, cardiac surgeons, interventional cardiologists, and primary care physicians.

53.3 Pearls

- Coronary CTA (CCTA) is an effective noninvasive test for the evaluation of patients with stable chest pain and suspected coronary artery disease (CAD). It is, however, a purely anatomical assessment, without functional information correlating to the sites of CAD.
- Fractional flow reserve (FFR) CT is the *noninvasive mathematically derived assessment computed from simulated pressure, velocity, and blood flow information obtained from static CT images in a CCTA.*
- FFR CT should be performed at the discretion of the interpreting radiologist taking into account feasibility (no motion artifacts) and degree of stenoses (at least one stenosis > 30%).
- Not every CT acquisition is suited for FFR calculation, mostly due to motion artifacts. These may be corrected prospectively by lowering patient's heart rate or retrospectively

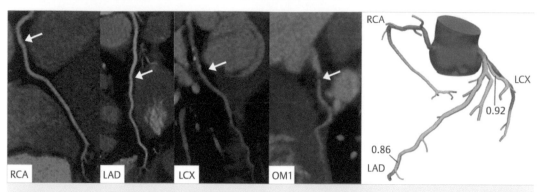

Fig. 53.1 Noncalcified plaques in the proximal LAD and RCA causing mild stenosis. LCX with mixed plaque proximally. Moderate stenosis noted in the proximal OM1 with a noncalcified atherosclerotic plaque. All fractional flow reserve (FFR) computed tomography (CT) results higher than 0.80 showing no hemodynamically significant stenoses in all vessels. LAD, left anterior descending artery; LCX, left circumflex artery; OM1, first obtuse marginal artery; RCA, right coronary artery.

Table 53.1 FFR CT reference values and interpretation

FFR CT reference values	
≥ 0.80	Low likelihood of flow-limitation requiring revascularization
0.75–0.79	Borderline value for flow-limitation requiring revascularization
< 0.75	High likelihood of flow-limitation requiring revascularization

Abbreviations: CT, computed tomography; FFR, fractional flow reserve.

by the use of thinner CT slices, by reconstructing additional series of the cardiac cycle.

- *FFR CT cannot be calculated in patients after bypass or in stented vessels.* The nonstented vessels can be still evaluated by FFR, except if stents are present in two different vessels or in the left main coronary.
- The first step in the interpretation of FFR CT is to re-examine the original coronary CTA study with particular focus on the location and severity of detailed anatomic lesions (▶ Fig. 53.1).
- FFR CT obtained up to 10 to 20 mm distal to the lower border of the stenosis will reflect the hemodynamic significance of that narrowing and should be used for decision making. CT FFR results can also be sampled at any point along

the vessels when the diameter of the sampled vessel is > 1.8 mm.

- The normal FFR CT cutoff is 0.80 or higher, considered borderline for anything between 0.75 and 0.79 and abnormal below 0.75 (▶ Table 53.1).
- Presence of mildly decreased FFR CT results (0.75–0.79) at the very distal aspect of the vessel might reflect alternative causes other than a single atherosclerotic plaque such as diffuse atherosclerotic disease along the vessel.
- FFR CT of 0.80 or less (▶ Fig. 53.2, ▶ Fig. 53.3, and ▶ Fig. 53.4) is a predictor of long-term clinical outcomes and is superior compared to the finding of clinically significant stenosis on coronary CT angiograms.
- A dichotomous interpretation strategy for clinical decision-making is to be considered only in lesions with FFR CT > 0.80 or ≤ 0.75, whereas, in patients with FFR CT ranging between 0.76 and 0.80 additional risk stratification information is needed.
- Patient symptoms, coronary anatomy, and suitability of revascularization should be reviewed in conjunction with FFR CT results.
- Normal FFR CT is associated with favorable long-term prognosis and the numeric value of FFR CT demonstrated an independent and inversely related risk continuum with clinical outcomes.

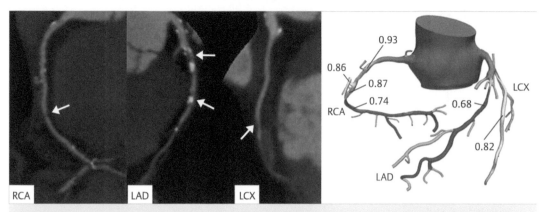

Fig. 53.2 Noncalcified atherosclerotic plaque in the mid RCA and diffuse mixed atherosclerotic plaque in the LAD causing moderate and severe stenosis, respectively, both with corresponding fractional flow reserve (FFR) computed tomography (CT) results lower than 0.80 indicating hemodynamical significance. Noncalcified atherosclerotic plaques in the mid LCX with normal FFR values. LAD, left anterior descending artery; LCX, left circumflex artery; RCA, right coronary artery.

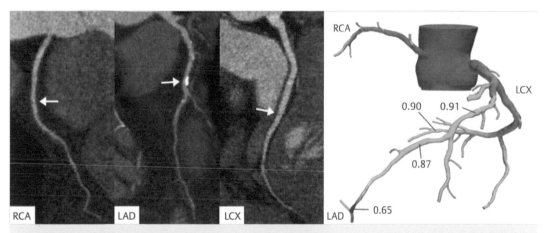

Fig. 53.3 Noncalcified atherosclerotic plaques in the proximal RCA and mid LCX causing mild stenoses with normal fractional flow reserve (FFR) values. Diffuse mixed atherosclerotic plaques in the proximal and mid LAD with no corresponding drop in FFR values. Abnormal FFR values are, however, noted in the more distal LAD, representing hemodynamically significant lower functional reserve with no specific single culprit lesion. LAD, left anterior descending artery; LCX, left circumflex artery; RCA, right coronary artery.

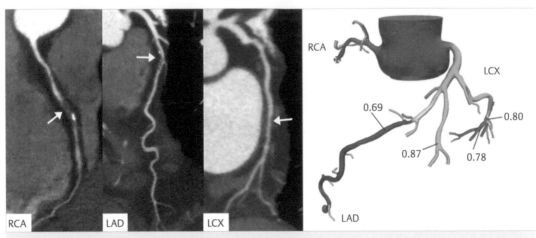

Fig. 53.4 Large noncalcified atherosclerotic plaque in the proximal RCA causing occlusion, confirmed in fractional flow reserve (FFR) evaluation. Mixed atherosclerotic plaque in the proximal LAD with immediate FFR value of 0.69, representing a hemodynamically significant stenosis. Noncalcified atherosclerotic plaque in the mid LCX with normal associate FFR value of 0.80. LAD, left anterior descending artery; LCX, left circumflex artery; RCA, right coronary artery.

Suggested Readings

Fairbairn TA, Nieman K, Akasaka T, et al. Real-world clinical utility and impact on clinical decision-making of coronary computed tomography angiography-derived fractional flow reserve: lessons from the ADVANCE Registry. Eur Heart J. 2018; 39 (41):3701–3711

Ihdayhid AR, Norgaard BL, Gaur S, et al. Prognostic value and risk continuum of noninvasive fractional flow reserve derived from coronary CT angiography. Radiology. 2019; 292(2):343–351

Liu X, Wang Y, Zhang H, et al. Evaluation of fractional flow reserve in patients with stable angina: can CT compete with angiography? Eur Radiol. 2019; 29(7):3669–3677

Nørgaard BL, Fairbairn TA, Safian RD, et al. Angiography derived fractional flow reserve testing in patients with stable coronary artery disease: recommendations on interpretation and reporting. Radiology: Cardiothorac Imag. 2019; 1(5)

Patel MR, Nørgaard BL, Fairbairn TA, et al. 1-Year impact on medical practice and clinical outcomes of FFRCT: the ADVANCE registry. JACC Cardiovasc Imaging. 2020; 13(1 Pt 1):97–105

Pontone G, Weir-McCall JR, Baggiano A, et al. Determinants of rejection rate for coronary CT angiography fractional flow reserve analysis. Radiology. 2019; 292(3):597–605

Index